THE PERFORMANCE NUTRITIONIST

Insights, reflections and advice
from practitioners working in elite sport

DR JAMES C. MOREHEN

Copyright © 2021 by Dr James C Morehen. All rights reserved.

This book or any portion thereof may not be reproduced or used in any manner whatsoever without the express written permission of the publisher except for the use of brief quotations in a book review.

Cover image by: U.T Designs
Book design by: SWATT Books Ltd

Printed in the United Kingdom
First Printing, 2021

ISBN: 978-1-7398718-0-2 (Paperback)
ISBN: 978-1-7398718-1-9 (eBook)

Dr James C Morehen
Bicester, Oxforshire

morehenperformance.com

CONTENTS

Acknowledgements — 5
Dedication — 7
Foreword — 9
Introduction — 11

CHAPTER 1: Craig Umenyi — 21

CHAPTER 2: Lloyd Parker — 33

CHAPTER 3: Dr Daniel Martin — 51

CHAPTER 4: Hannah Sheridan — 65

CHAPTER 5: Dr Marcus Hannon — 81

CHAPTER 6: Dr Emma Tester — 93

CHAPTER 7: Dr Jill Leckey — 107

CHAPTER 8: Dr Chris Rosimus — 121

CHAPTER 9: Emma Gardner — 133

CHAPTER 10:	Professor James Morton	*149*
CONCLUSION:	How to stand out from the crowd	*167*
	Find out more about	
	Morehen Performance Mentorship	*173*
	Praise for Morehen Performance Mentorship	*175*
	Keep in touch	*179*
	References	*181*
	About the author	*185*

ACKNOWLEDGEMENTS

Thank you to the many students and nutritionists who reached out to me personally via social media channels and inspired me to start this project in the first place. It was because of you, and my own experiences navigating my career, that this book is now in your hands.

I would like to say a personal thank you to the 10 performance nutritionists who I interviewed for this book. Without you kindly agreeing to spend your time with me, this book simply would not have come to fruition. The knowledge, insights and honest advice you openly share will inspire practitioners who read this book to become better at the delivery of performance nutrition to the elite performers we all work with.

Finally, thank you to Karen, Louise and Sam for your support to get this book over the line and published. Without your guidance it would not have been possible.

DEDICATION

I dedicate this book to Nura and our first child, my mum, my brothers and of course my dad.

Remember, today is the tomorrow you worried about yesterday.

FOREWORD

As an undergraduate student, my favourite textbook was the classic *Exercise Physiology: Nutrition, Energy and Human Performance*, authored by McArdle, Katch and Katch. In addition to being an outstanding text, several chapters were preceded by an interview with a world-leading expert from our field. I would often lie in bed each night, reading and re-reading the words of wisdom and advice from some of the founding figures of sport and exercise science. With a rapidly growing interest in exercise metabolism, the interviews with Professors Dave Costill, John Holloszy and Bengt Saltin were standouts for me. Their words would encourage me to approach the laboratory the next day with a sense of curiosity, rigour and attention to detail, essential ingredients that are required for life as a researcher.

When I soon realised that the applied extension of human metabolism was performance nutrition, I naturally looked for other mentors from which to draw life lessons and sources of inspiration. I managed to find one such interview with Professor Louise Burke, published in the *International Journal of Sports Nutrition and Exercise Metabolism* in 2009. Louise outlined how her career in sport nutrition essentially began with writing a letter to the star player of her favourite Australian Football team, the result of which was the club doctor inviting her to the club to "help out". Thankfully, as my career progressed, I managed to surround myself with experts and mentors from all round the world (including Louise herself), all of whom have shaped my practice in one way or another. My journey as a practitioner also began with people welcoming a stranger into their environment, that being a local amateur boxing club in Liverpool. Within weeks of walking through the gym door, I was soon helping both amateur and professional fighters "make weight" for contests, learning my trade whilst travelling around the country to and from boxing shows. Closer to home, myself and trusted friend, Professor Graeme Close, began to share an office (and still do to this day), allowing us to debate all aspects of applied practice on a daily basis. In setting up the MSc course in Sport Nutrition at Liverpool John Moores University, we soon had a flow of eager-to-learn students coming to our office each day. Our conversations were deeper and richer than ever before and as students became entrenched in their placement module, we frequently discussed our "tales from the field" in the classroom each week.

Aside from technical knowledge, I quickly learned that we are in the people profession and that the role of the performance nutritionist is to therefore positively impact people. My reflections have taught me that it is just as important to learn from your own and others' experiences as it is to learn the biochemical steps of glycolysis. For this reason, I am delighted to author the foreword for *The Performance Nutritionist*, a text that presents a series of reflections from early to mid-career practitioners. I hope you enjoy reading these pages as much as I did.

I am frequently humbled by the fact that people ask me for advice on a career as a researcher and practitioner. However, as I approach my 40th birthday, I readily acknowledge that I have much still to learn. As such, I will continue to do what I have always done. I will surround myself with mentors and people with superior skillsets and experience than myself. I will surround myself with people who support and challenge me to be better. In reading *The Performance Nutritionist*, I hope that this text will encourage you to do the same.

Stay hungry,
James Morton, November 2021

INTRODUCTION

There are 85 universities in the UK which offer degree courses related to sport science and/or nutrition. Multiply these 85 institutes by 35 – the mean student cohort group per year group (which, by the way, is substantially lower than my year group at Liverpool John Moores University of 300!) – and this gives you about 3000 students each year.

Every year, around 3000 sport and exercise science students throw their mortarboard caps up in the air at the graduation ceremony marking the end of their degree programme. This throw signals the end of the degree and then the start of the dog-eat-dog hunt to go and get a full-time role working in elite sport with professional athletes.

However, there is an issue. There simply aren't enough jobs for the number of students who want to work in this industry. OK, not all of those who graduate will want to get into sport or nutrition related fields, but a good number would love to. Using an example to highlight the issue, in the UK there are 96 football teams in the top tiers of English football, 24 rugby teams in the top two tiers of professional rugby union and 12 rugby league teams in the top division in rugby league. If each one of these teams employed a full-time nutritionist, then this would allow 132 nutritionists to be employed. I know there are many other sports you can work in as a nutritionist, but I'm sure you can see the point I am making. Lots of students seeking employment, but not many jobs.

It's a common issue my colleagues and I hear each year: new graduates saying that they have finished their degree programme, they have a 2:1 or a first-class honours in sport science and/or nutrition, but every time they apply for a job, they either don't get an interview, or if they do, they don't get offered the job. They have been beaten to it by someone else.

What's the main issue and problem then? A lot of the time "experience" crops up as the reason that people are not successful with a job application. Have you ever gone through a job interview and felt like you have done well, only to be called or emailed to say you just did not have enough experience compared to other practitioners? Have you completed a degree in sport science but don't have the physical knowledge and experience of working with athletes?

We have all been there. I was twice! The first time this happened to me was when I applied for a director of sport nutrition role at an American university. I was told someone else had more experience than me. The second time was when I applied for a role at a Premiership football club. They didn't even reply to my application, and my next job application had a negative result. It was time to look in the mirror and self-reflect. I asked myself what I was missing. I realised I needed more experience.

If you've already got experience of working with athletes, then you may be battling with the decision of whether you need to complete a master's or even PhD to progress forward on the journey to your dream job role. This is another common question that I see many students ask on online conferences or in classrooms where I teach.

Surely then, you want to know what the key traits are of performance nutritionists who are currently working at the elite level of sport? What can you learn from people in the industry currently that will help you either gain experience or be successful in your next job application?

Wouldn't it be nice to know what some of the biggest challenges were that respected practitioners have faced in their careers to date, and importantly how they navigated their way around them? Well, that is exactly what this book will uncover.

Over the last 18 months I have interviewed 10 well-respected nutritionists, including applied researchers, doctors and a professor, asked them key questions and teased out brilliant answers which will help you improve your own chances of being successful in your career.

Before we get into the main part of the book and I tell you more about the people I interviewed, I think it's fitting to share my own career to date, so you know more about me and why I have created this book. I have been (and still am) fortunate to work alongside genuine world-leading researchers and practitioners within applied physiology and sport nutrition.

Between the ages of 18 and 21, I had no ambition to study at university. I moved to Mont Tremblant in Quebec, Canada and for two winter seasons trained as a professional snowboard instructor. In the summers I came back to the UK, worked in Pizza Hut full time as a waiter, saved up my tips and then flew to Southeast Asia to travel around Thailand, Cambodia and Vietnam. I did this for three years and loved it. At 21 years old, I had "matured" and was ready to go to university to study.

If I am honest, like most sport science students I grew up wanting to be a professional athlete. I wasn't dedicated enough as a teenager and my rugby skills were not as good as others at my age. Once I was old enough to go out and party, this also took over and my rugby training took a back seat. Knowing that I was never going to "make it" as a professional athlete, I knew that I wanted to work with professional athletes as a career. Researching online and speaking to people at career fairs, it was obvious I needed to study a degree in a sport related area.

I moved to Liverpool to start my undergraduate degree in Sport and Exercise Science at the world-leading institute, Liverpool John Moores University (LJMU). I loved the course, and the city was amazing. During my final undergraduate year, I had my first exposure to assisting with professional athletes. A PhD student at the time, the now Dr George Wilson was completing his research projects with professional jockeys, and I asked him if I could help and assist in data collection. He agreed and this was the start of my applied experience.

After my undergraduate studies, it was a no-brainer for me to stay at LJMU and so I started my MSc in Sport Physiology. This was a year-long course which was difficult and enjoyable. I failed one of the modules and had to resit it which meant I could only get a pass grade of 40% and therefore this pulled down my overall grade to about 62% (a merit).

During this year, my applied placement module on my course was helping the St Helens Rugby League team in the university altitude chamber. Every Wednesday morning, I would wake up at 6am and walk to university to switch it on. At 7am, injured rugby players would arrive with the club performance staff and they would use the altitude chamber to perform off-feet aerobic conditioning with the players. Although this placement was only meant to last for six weeks, I wanted to carry on gaining this experience with elite athletes, so I asked if the performance staff would like to carry on using the chamber, which of course they said they would love to do. We continued the Wednesday morning altitude chamber session for the rest of the season.

Using my initiative, I asked the performance staff if it would be possible to come into the club every Saturday morning to assist with sport science support with the players. I didn't mind what I did, I just wanted to be in and around the environment. They agreed. So during this year, every Saturday morning I would wake up at 5.45am for the 45-minute cycle and train ride to their training facility. Although I was shattered and in the winter months it was pitch black outside, I loved it and I was gaining invaluable experience volunteering each Wednesday and Saturday with professional rugby players, which carried on until I graduated with my MSc degree.

After this experience, I asked the captain of the club and head of strength and conditioning if they would supply me with a reference. They did. I then sent these to Saracens Rugby Club along with a cover letter to ask if I would be able to pop into their club over the summer months – as it was the closest premiership rugby club to my parents' home. They agreed and I then started a summer placement with the academy team, assisting with whatever they needed me to do. I had to drive the 90 minutes from Colchester to St Albans three times per week, spending about £150 a week on petrol. At the end of this period, my bank balance was negative, but I had gained an enormous amount of invaluable experience.

Whilst studying my master's at LJMU, I enjoyed the research and applied practice so much that I had a feeling that the next step in my career was to study a PhD. But not any old PhD; it had to be one that was going to give me even more experience working with professional athletes. So, I had many meetings with both Professors James Morton and Graeme Close to ask them what opportunities they had, if they knew of any PhDs looming, and what it actually entailed. They advised me to speak to a few of the current PhD students at the university, individuals like (now) Dr Sam Impey, Dr Jon Bartlett and Dr Carl Langan-Evans. So, I had coffees with all three of them and peppered them with fact-finding questions about their PhDs, their thoughts on PhDs and their advice if I were to do one.

Following these discussions, it was clear that a PhD was what I wanted to do. I was happy and ready to commit to another three years of higher education and become a mini-expert in my area of study. Now I needed to either find the money for a PhD or apply for one with funding.

Not many people are aware that I applied for a PhD at LJMU which was fully funded and with Kevin Keegan (the ex-England football manager's company). It involved studying young football players and the effectiveness of a football simulator on makers of health (i.e. increased fitness and improved body composition). I was successful in my application, and they offered me the PhD. Happy days, I was ready to start.

However, after thinking about it over the weekend, and reflecting on my conversations with the current PhD students, I knew that I needed to be 100% certain that I was passionate about this study area as I would be researching this area for the next three years of my life. The simple answer was no, this was not the PhD for me to study. On Monday morning I politely declined the offer and explained my reasons. Back to square one. You may think I was bonkers, but I couldn't commit to it fully because my passion was not going to be there.

Fast forward a few months and along came the lucky break I was waiting for. Graeme Close had an opportunity for me to do a fully funded PhD in collaboration with a professional rugby league team and the university. Amazing! This was the one for me.

For the next 4½ years of my career I studied my PhD full time and worked full time as the performance nutritionist embedded within two professional rugby league teams. In the first year it was Widnes Vikings and then I moved to Warrington Wolves where we successfully won the league and made two cup finals in my first season.

It was during this time that I really built up my craft knowledge as a practitioner, working in the club during the day as a performance nutritionist and then reading and learning in the evening (when I wasn't too tired, or in the pub!). I was fortunate that my four PhD publications were completed with professional players as my participants and published in peer-reviewed, well-respected journals.

The reason my PhD took 4½ years to complete instead of the traditional three years full time was mainly due to the heavy time commitments that I had at each of the clubs during the day. It was difficult to manage sometimes, and on reflection I didn't manage it as well as I should have.

One of the other reasons that I wanted to study a PhD was to do my dad proud. But unfortunately, he never saw me graduate as a doctor. On the 20th October 2019 I received a phone call from my older brother to inform me that our dad had had a fatal cardiac arrest. Nothing could have been done; it was lights out and goodbye. The reason I tell this part of my journey is because everyone has their ups and downs in their life. This was a seriously low part of my journey and a period of my life that I will never forget.

Following Dad's death, I spent some time at home with the family and in particular my mum to support them all. When I was ready, I went back to Liverpool and decided that enough was enough; it was time to really dial in, focus and get the PhD done. I wanted to do my PhD viva on my dad's birthday, the 17th April, and so this was the target date. Graeme was outstanding in his support over the next six months, and I owe him tremendously for how he guided me to the finish line. I handed the PhD in at the beginning of March, completed my viva on the date planned with Dad watching over me, and graduated that summer a doctor.

My thesis was entitled "Growing, Building and Repairing Elite Rugby Players: Nutritional and Energetic Considerations". It was one of the proudest moments of my life and my mother, brothers and partner were with me to support and celebrate. With eight publications to my name and a Silver award from the Gatorade Sport Science Institute at the European Congress of Sport Science for my final PhD study, I can say I am happy and proud of my academic journey.

Now the PhD was complete, it was time to get a "real" job and work full time within professional sport. I was made aware of a job advert for a performance nutritionist at The Football Association working for England football. Although football is not my passion, I thought I would apply for it anyway to see if I would get an interview. About 85 people applied for the role globally; I made the final 12 who had a phone call with the head of performance. This went well and I made the final cut of six people who were invited to St George's Park (the home of the England football training centre) for face-to-face interviews. I was successful with the interview and so started a four-year journey with England football.

Although this was great and an enjoyable role, I always felt like I was in third gear in terms of what I was able to deliver and achieve at the FA. This wasn't anyone's fault; the structure of how international football operates didn't give me the job satisfaction that I needed. As such, I handed my notice in and started a new role as Head of Nutrition with Bristol Bears, a rugby union team in the premiership division.

Throughout my master's, PhD and even now, I have also enjoyed the odd project here and there with professional athletes, corporate clients and the weekend warrior. I have always said yes. This has allowed me to work in Premiership football, rugby league, with professional boxers, combat sport athletes and Formula 1, 2 and 3 drivers, and successfully launch my own performance consultancy business.

So I've come from being an 18-year-old snowboarder in Canada to a performance nutritionist working in professional sport, and I reflect on my short career so far with fond memories. I'm not done yet; I have a clear vison of where I want to get to next on my own career path and am more motivated than ever to achieve my goals.

I hope after reading this section you are motivated too. This book is for you if you want help to achieve your goals. If you are currently studying and want to get ahead of the curve, then read the chapters and take notes of key areas you think you can improve on before you finish your degree.

And if...

- You have finished your undergraduate degree and want to get your first job but have not been successful with job applications yet
- You are struggling to get experience with athletes and access to working with athletes
- You have finished your master's degree programme, you have great knowledge but lack the transferable skills to now go and apply the knowledge
- You find yourself in an interview and look good on paper but crumble when in the interview

... then get stuck in and read on.

You will learn how 10 well-respected researchers and practitioners have navigated their own way into working at the elite end of professional sport. You will find out how they got their jobs and discover more about their journey and progress in their careers – including the mistakes they have made so that you can avoid them.

We talk about the key characteristics that are essential to become a successful nutritionist.

Their interviews are full of golden nuggets of information and tips which they have learnt over their careers to date. They provide advice on key actions and areas to develop which you can be doing now to help you get the dream job you want once you have graduated.

Here are the 10 people I interviewed for this book:

1. Craig Umenyi – Performance nutritionist, formerly Tottenham Hotspur Football Club
2. Lloyd Parker – Everton Football Club

3. Dr Daniel Martin – Southampton Football Club, Haas Formula 1, Professional Jockeys
4. Hannah Sheridan – Tottenham Hotspur Football Club
5. Dr Marcus Hannon – Aston Villa Football Club
6. Dr Emma Tester – Tottenham Hotspur Football Club, formerly Munster Rugby Union
7. Dr Jill Leckey – Australian Cycling Team
8. Dr Chris Rosimus – England football
9. Emma Gardner – England Cricket, Great Britain Hockey
10. Professor James Morton – Professor of Exercise Metabolism, Director of Performance Solutions at Science in Sport, the FA and Premier League High-Performance Mentor

As you read these chapters I would like you to reflect on key areas that stand out for you and how you can apply the learning from these moments in your own career. Having personally interviewed everyone myself, I have learnt from each person and applied their golden nuggets of advice and lessons into my own practice. Let's get stuck into the first interview with Craig.

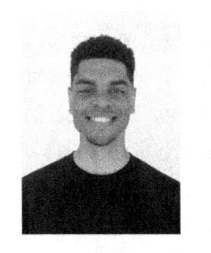

CHAPTER 1:
CRAIG UMENYI

Craig worked as the first team nutritionist at Tottenham Hotspur Football Club and Arsenal Football Club. Craig has worked as a performance nutritionist for five years and previously studied his undergraduate degree at Kingston University in Sport Science with Business and his Master's degree in Sports Nutrition at Liverpool John Moores University.

I was studying for my PhD at Liverpool John Moores University when Craig started his MSc there. He asked to have a coffee with me and ask me a few questions about my experience working with Widnes Vikings and Warrington Wolves rugby teams. Having just started his role with Toronto Wolfpack, he was keen to bounce some ideas around with me. Since then, we have stayed close friends and have shared experiences and stories with each other.

You can follow Craig on Twitter at @CraigUmenyi

Craig, the purpose of this book is to help aspiring performance nutritionists to break into the industry and learn from people like yourself and your experiences. To kick it off, please can you introduce yourself. Who are you and what is your background? Additionally, how did you get into nutrition in the first place?[1]

Craig: I am a performance nutritionist, having previously worked in Premier League football. I began like a lot of sports nutritionists, doing a sport science degree. At the end of the degree, I had developed my interest in sports performance. To be honest, I didn't really know what to do and how that would translate to a career, or even what specific field that I wanted to go down. I took some time out; it wasn't intentional, but sometimes these things just happen and fall into place. Therefore, I decided to take a year away from studying and worked as a travel agent.

About three years went by and I kept telling myself that the following September I would be doing a master's somewhere. I kept putting it off every year for different reasons. For example, one year it was because I didn't have enough money, the next year it was just that I liked my current situation, or the course that I wanted to do fell through. I then started the International Society of Sports Nutrition (ISSN) diploma. During that time, I still tried to read new research. I started helping a friend of mine who worked with a young racing driver just doing food diaries and dietary analysis for a tenner – really basic stuff, to be honest!

I was in a job which wasn't inspiring or energising me, therefore I started to do the diploma. I was quite fortunate; I was living at home at the time and had spent all my savings on the diploma. I'm grateful for my parents who told me not to worry about paying rent. They said to put my money into the course. I got started with the course and really enjoyed it.

I got to the point of needing to think about how the course may open up some opportunities for me. With this in mind, I wanted to develop further and came across the sports nutrition course at LJMU. I applied for it and got accepted. I moved to Liverpool and really enjoyed the course, the work placements etc. Fortunately enough, following the course I went

---

1   My questions and comments are in bold throughout the interview chapters.

immediately into a role at Arsenal Football Club within the academy as the performance nutritionist three days a week and from there it just kind of unfolded. That role went to a full-time role the following season, before I took my current role at Tottenham Hotspurs. That's my journey, which with the four-year gap between studying and different jobs, is probably a bit unconventional, but it taught me patience.

So just going back to the master's degree at LJMU then, was it the year after that you then applied for the role at Arsenal Football Club? Also were you successful straight away or did you have a period of job hunting?

Craig: I was one of that 0.05% who are very fortunate to go straight into work. I was ridiculously fortunate. The job advert went live towards the end of studying at LJMU and I was grateful to have Professor Graeme Close and Dr Marcus Hannon to use as referees from when I did my work placement with them at Everton Football Club. I literally moved out of my place in Liverpool and the next day was back in London and working at Arsenal Football Club.

That is a quick transition in our industry. How did you prepare for such a quick change?

Craig: One thing that helped prepare me for the role was the 3–4 years I had away from education, especially the 12–18-month period before enrolling on the MSc programme. In this period, I started to do meal plans or dietary analysis and gave basic nutrition advice for minimal payment. By the time I had finished at LJMU I felt confident to call myself a performance nutritionist.

I'm not sure if it's just me, but there's almost a breaking point where one day you feel confident enough to call yourself a performance nutritionist which I probably shied away from until someone actually paid me. Being exposed to other working environments helped greatly – so I wasn't taken aback as much when I was in some of these sporting environments. For sure, the knowledge and insight gained from the MSc programme and the work placement experiences were vital in helping me develop, although I do recognise that time away working in totally unrelated industries from education and sport helped me approach my time at LJMU differently and feel more comfortable in the interview process.

I agree with you, experience and building craft knowledge is key for our industry. As you reflect on your career to date, who are some of your biggest mentors that you would look back on and think they have a key influence in your career? Additionally, why have they been so important to you?

Craig: Studying at LJMU, Professors Graeme Close and James Morton were a huge influence. James is incredibly reflective, which as I've matured personally and professionally, I recognise the importance of each year. What I took from Graeme is that you can be very successful in this industry by leaning into your natural personality and being yourself. To see someone who has been successful, has numerous academic publications and isn't afraid to try new avenues and ventures, is admirable. From the outside looking in, I did think that to work in sport you had to be a certain way, not show too much of your personality and almost conform to the norm. There are environments that I have been in that encourage that and I think it can be easy to lose yourself.

Ultimately both James and Graeme drove home the importance of building relationships and remembering that we are in the industry of working with people. Of course, the nutrition knowledge is fundamental but when you're working in sporting environments people skills are paramount. It's also about learning to build and tolerate relationships with difficult people; that's the reality of professional sport.

As you full well know, although sport nutrition is a growing industry, it's quite a small industry at the same time. With this, bouncing ideas off other practitioners is important. I always come away from interactions with David Dunne having food for thought and breaking away from convention. Likewise with yourself, James. I did some work with Dr Marcus Hannon for a year and that really changed my outlook on some of the research that he's done in terms of working with youth athletes. This really helped my role with academy football players.

There is a key lesson here, to utilise those around you and those you respect in the industry. After all, if they are your friends then even better.

With your career to date, is there a standout moment for you? Is there something that springs to mind that you'd be comfortable sharing?

Craig: It may sound a little bit cheesy, but I'd say leaving Arsenal Football Club was something that really stood out for me. You know what it's like in sport, a lot of the time we don't get nice goodbyes. We have all heard stories of people who get shown the back door and you don't get to have the send-off that you should have had, the respect and courtesy that your work and time deserves.

When I left Arsenal Football Club, my department manager, Des Ryan, the U18s, U23s players and staff gave me a really nice farewell and an opportunity to speak and have the space to directly hear from players about the impact that I had on them. The pace of the job moves so fast that you don't think about these moments, but they stick in the mind of athletes. Coming back to the aspect of building relationships, it was a big moment for me to have a send-off like that. To know I had built relationships with people and to maintain those with players and staff even now is important to me.

Nice reflection. As you reflect on your career again, is there a standout moment that was a challenge for you?

Craig: Whenever you go into a new environment there's always a little bit of self-doubt as you try to suss out the environment. You know you have to build relationships, whilst there's also the pressure of being seen to have an immediate impact.

When I joined Arsenal Football Club, the role came with a level of responsibility and accountability. It was a new process for me and there was an element of impostor syndrome. You look around and you think everyone else is really on their "A game" but after about a few months you realise that you're there for a reason too.

When I reflect on moving on to Tottenham Hotspurs, I entered an environment with a team that was already very successful; they had just been in a Champions League final. The department was full of experienced practitioners that have been a part of and helped build the current nutrition department. Being in this environment gets you to think about what innovative ideas you are going to bring to the club and not just change things for the sake of changing them. I used to ask myself, how do you work with world class players who may have egos? When you're working at this level you also deal with staff who have egos, so again it's a different set of challenges. It's human to have a little bit of doubt going into a new environment as a sports nutritionist, especially as there can be a pressure to make visible changes immediately.

You previously mentioned staying true to yourself and being authentic was key. What other characteristics do you think people need to work in the industry of performance nutrition?

Craig: When I studied at LJMU, I was working with Toronto Wolfpack, a rugby league team. I think the transition from the rugby league environment, with predominantly northern lads, with lots of banter, was a whole new world. Compare this to a London-based football academy with an ethnically and culturally diverse population which was a lot more similar to me and the environment I grew up in.

I probably gained the respect of the rugby league players because I wasn't trying to mirror who they naturally are. I've never played rugby, so I think going in and being true to yourself whilst also demonstrating that you want to learn more about the culture and listening to people was hugely important. People connect with people, so I found that although rugby league wasn't the most comfortable environment for me to work in initially, after a while they just respected me for who I was and liked that I made an effort to learn. Of course, if you've got some credibility and some knowledge that will help too. It can be a difficult one, and again it can be very easy to be a little bit swayed to change who you are. You and I spoke about how work environments and different organisations can have an effect on you, but ultimately you have to recognise who you are. I have always found athletes to be incredible at detecting support staff who aren't genuine.

Definitely. I have so many reflections on my own transition from rugby league into international football which I have learned so much from. One of the reasons I have written this book is to allow those aspiring nutritionists to learn from you and your journey. Hypothetically, if there was a five years younger Craig, ringing the Craig that I'm talking to now, is there anything you would advise that individual?

Craig: I would say to always work on your people skills and exposing yourself to different people and environments. My path to working in sport wasn't necessarily conventional. I worked in different fields in different industries around different people; very few of my friends worked or had an interest in sport. I think from that aspect, I didn't have the same tunnel vision that maybe sometimes you can experience if education and/or sport is all that you've ever really known.

If you want to work in sport you are going to be in environments when you maybe don't see eye to eye with others or people don't fully respect or appreciate nutrition. It's going to be uncomfortable because for the most part we are under-recognised and under-appreciated. As practitioners, we love the athlete that is 100% adherent and interested in every intervention we suggest, but you're going to work with many who are not. Can you be adaptable to condense or prioritise the key areas for them to focus on and regularly check in on them?

I think that's a massive area that young students now need to learn quickly. The enjoyment of being comfortable with being vulnerable. A recent book I read by Brené Brown (*Daring Greatly*) was about how it is fine to be vulnerable in situations and to bring your personality. In my opinion, personality pleases people. People want to see a personality, and this lends itself to the next area that I want to talk about. Most master's degree programmes in sports nutrition include the academic and fundamental knowledge, however is there anything that you didn't learn on course that you think is important if you're going to be a successful practitioner working in professional sport?

Craig: Of course, the nutritional knowledge is fundamental, but I think we have become too focused with things like carbohydrate-periodising meal plans and probably not enough on how effective we can be when we need to work with people. For example, does the athlete actually listen? Can you encourage them do something different to what they are used to? Better yet, can you step out of your own biases and beliefs around food and nutrition to meet them with their beliefs even if it's not "best practice"?

There aren't many people in the world that don't know what good food would look like; it's quite easy to distinguish a bad diet and a good diet. However, I think there is an element of how well we as practitioners can educate our athletes and what they should be doing instead of what they should not be doing.

Craig: Absolutely. As nutritionists, like everybody else, we come with our own biases and preferences regarding food. As a result, this may limit the effectiveness of your practice when you're trying to get people to see food through the same lenses that you see it through. At some point in your career, you may have worked with an overweight person who may have grown up as an overweight child and as such their relationship with food is very different to the lean football player who's been able to eat everything and has never had to worry about fat mass gain. Additionally, factors like nationalities, family backgrounds, ethnicity can affect views on food. Sometimes we may force people into our view of food and when they don't agree, we struggle to communicate the message or dismiss the athlete as being difficult, when really, we as practitioners aren't understanding the athlete fully.

Where do you think the future of performance nutrition will be in five years' time?

Craig: As an industry, I do not see there being a greater abundance of professional jobs any more than current numbers. There are only a finite number of teams and resources. I think it's more about how people become more entrepreneurial to deliver nutrition to more people. This might be a semi-pro athlete; it might be the weekend warriors. To be a performance nutritionist, I think people should consider the journey and requirements a little bit more.

I was one of those people, like most students, studying a master's in sports nutrition and was able to do a placement at a football team. In this moment, you're probably not thinking about working with the 45-year-old who likes to cycle at the weekend for fun. Of course, that's not your dream, but I think to recognise there are other avenues of profitable work is important. I think we'll start to recognise and appreciate the human aspect regarding food more – emotions, behaviour, environment etc.

Have you recently read a book that you would recommend to others in the industry?

Craig: I also read *Daring Greatly* by Brené Brown a few months ago and that jumped out at me for a lot of things. You already alluded to being vulnerable. Recognising that everyone has their own vulnerabilities and not shying away from yours. In doing so, you feel freer to be bold and daring rather than simply staying small and playing safe. It was a very useful book. In the professional setting I couldn't always figure out why people acted in a certain way. As I got older and after reading this book, I realised it is individuals' defence mechanisms, insecurities, and the need to maintain a certain image or persona.

Moving on, are there any key principles that you try to follow every day that keep you on the straight and narrow?

Craig: I haven't been the most disciplined with exercise, however running outdoors is great for me. I try to find small pockets of time to daydream ideas and write them down. I think trying to find creative options is important – I often use cooking as a method for this. It's important to have a life and quality relationships with others outside of this work, otherwise it is too easy to become consumed by it. I used to be one of those people who would read academic research, almost obsessive with wanting more knowledge all the time. However, more recently I read books in all different areas of life, and this makes me happier.

Finally, in your opinion, what makes us a successful performance nutritionist?

Craig: Being proactive. That hasn't always been my biggest strength or skill set. I'm very fortunate to have worked previously with Hannah Sheridan at Tottenham Hotspurs. Something I took from Hannah is how important it is to do the smaller things and being able to do them consistently. Little reminders and nudges to keep people focused. Lastly, it is really important to show people that you care about them and to engage in conversations about them outside of nutrition and sport. This goes a long way to build a transparent and open relationship with individuals and athletes.

MY REFLECTIONS FROM CRAIG'S INTERVIEW

Craig is one of the few students who finished a course and got a job straight away. Having said this, it is clear how much Craig values being yourself, staying true to yourself and building meaningful relationships around you. It is important these extend outside of sport as well to ensure you do not become fully absorbed by work and lose the work-life balance.

This links in nicely to where Craig talks about respecting and valuing that each person comes from a different background and will have their own biases towards food and therefore nutrition.

My final sentence on this interview is how initially Craig did not know what he wanted to do at the end of his undergraduate, but through life experiences and taking time out to think about his career he then walked the path he has been on to date.

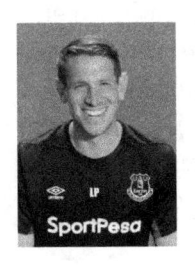

CHAPTER 2:
LLOYD PARKER

Lloyd is currently the Head of Nutrition at Everton Football Club and has been practising as a nutritionist for seven years.

He originally studied for an undergraduate degree in Sport Science at Brunel University before moving over to Hertfordshire to study another undergraduate degree in Dietetics, and is one of a small number of nutritionists in the industry with both degrees. Afterwards, Lloyd went to study for a MSc in Sport and Exercise Nutrition followed by a PhD at LJMU.

I first met Lloyd at LJMU in 2015 by way of introduction from Professor Graeme Close. At the time, I had recently started my PhD and Lloyd was working at Manchester City and was due to start his PhD with Everton. Both new to the PhD journey, we met up many times for a drink to share experiences from both our applied and PhD work. As Lloyd explains in our interview, the year he studied dietetics was a very important stage of his journey into both Manchester City Football Club and then Everton Football Club.

You can follow Lloyd on Twitter @parkernutrition

Could you give a bit of a background as to who you are and where you're working at the moment?

Lloyd: I currently work as the Head of Nutrition for Everton Football Club. My career started when I did a sport science undergraduate degree. I didn't know where to go afterwards and so I took a year out to travel. When I returned to my parents, they said to me, "Right, what are you going to do now you have had that time off?" I was already interested in nutrition before university because I had gained a lot of weight and I wanted to lose it, which I achieved successfully. Following this, my interest in nutrition developed. To study nutrition in the early 2000s was quite difficult; there weren't a huge number of courses or jobs around.

At the time, a lot of people told me to do a second degree and it's one of the best bits of advice that I received, and I did another undergraduate degree in dietetics. Although it meant my university life extended, it's benefited me in the long term. I probably wouldn't be where I am now without it.

Throughout the dietetics degree, I was also working in the National Health Service (NHS) for a couple years with weight management. It taught me a lot of stuff that I use today. A lot of behaviour change concepts for example. In the NHS, they cover behaviour change a lot and these concepts are like what you do with elite athletes. Nutritionists are trying to change behaviours and trying to change practice. Therefore, it doesn't really matter if you're working with someone who is 150kg and ready for bariatric surgery or if they are an elite athlete ready to play a football match. A lot of the time, it is the same principle.

After I finished my dietetics degree, I worked in the NHS for a few years. I knew the clinical side of nutrition well, but I didn't know enough of the sports nutrition side. Therefore, I did a postgraduate in sport and exercise nutrition at Coventry University, which was great as it bridged the gap between the sport science and clinical nutrition knowledge I had.

At that point I met a nice practitioner working at Warrington Wolves and she said that the academy rugby team needed some help. I therefore did some work with the Warrington Wolves Academy. I collected skinfold measurements for body fat assessments and presented in front of players and parents. Whilst I was at Warrington Wolves, I did the International Society for the Advancement of Kinanthropometry accreditation and met my now good friend, Shane Murphy, who was working at Manchester City Football Club. We got chatting and stayed in contact. Three months later, he called me and said, "Manchester City Academy are looking for a paid internship sports scientist role, but you'll be expected to do a lot of things. The main area needing focus on at the moment is nutrition."

Me and one other practitioner went for the interview, and I was extremely lucky because they went off word of mouth from people that they knew within the industry. I managed to secure the role.

I had a nice breadth of practice. I was doing gym sessions with the academy players, and I was collecting and downloading GPS. I was tasked with designing and implementing a nutrition strategy at the club because they had nothing previously. I did this for a year and then they employed me as a consultant to focus purely on nutrition. I also started to do some paid work with Salford Red Devils Rugby League team and started working at Manchester City Women's Team while they turned professional. This was a really exciting project as they had just bought some really big players, Steph Houghton who is the England captain, Jill Scott and Toni Duggan. This was my first chance to work in female sport.

About five years ago, I received a call from Professor Graeme Close who asked if I would like to work at Everton Football Club. My initial thoughts were "Wow, where has this come from?" It was 07:30 and I was in the gym. He replied and said we're going to speak to Everton Football Club, and we think you are a good person for the first team nutrition role. This meant there was no interview process, which was crazy considering the role. I spoke to the head of sport science at the club, and he said that he liked me and asked when could I start? My initial reaction was, well this is a bit of a whirlwind!

Graeme Close, Marcus Hannon (who is now working at Aston Villa Football Club) and I developed the team at Everton Football Club. It is a unique model, as often as nutritionists you are a bit of a lone wolf; there is normally only one of you. I think it's the only club in football where there were three of us working there together and we were able to build something special over a three-year cycle. Unfortunately, for the club, but fortunately for Marcus, he did well, he completed his PhD and then moved on. Therefore, we had to rebuild the model. We've now got another academy nutritionist who's working with the women's team, and we are now building the new department.

Amazing! A great path and journey. Rewinding a little, to confirm, your first role in nutrition was a blend of Warrington Wolves rugby and Manchester City Football Club?

Lloyd: I remind people all the time how I went on a whim with the Warrington gig. The lecturer at the time said she needed help and I think she thought that nobody would be interested. I lived in Liverpool at the time and the opportunity sounded great. I was really keen to work in sport. This keenness got me entry into the club.

For the Manchester City interview, I explained how I had worked with younger athletes before and how I had presented to parents and young athletes, and had set up a nutrition education pathway. Altogether, I think that's what got me the Manchester City role as well.

It all spiralled from me being keen. I was working full time in the NHS and would happily go to the rugby club for three hours in the evening two or three times a week. This was a key moment for me. Just go for it; if there's an opportunity, grab it with both hands and do everything you can to make the most of it.

I always think of these moments as a "jump and the net will catch you" moment.

Lloyd: Absolutely, people often said to me I was lucky. You must create your own luck and have some luck along the way. I mean I'm a big believer of the more opportunities you give yourself, the more luck you will receive.

Previously you mentioned a couple of names. These may be your mentors, or they may not, but who are the key people in your career and why have they been so important for you?

Lloyd: I think these people change and evolve as you progress along your career and some people might be there for a snapshot. When I was debating what to do at the start of my career, my mum's friend rang me up and recommended I did dietetics. She said that it would help get my career off to a good start. So, although she hasn't been a long-standing mentor so to speak, she was a really key person in my life at that time to direct me down that path.

Professor Graeme Close has been great for me. He is always at the end of the phone, and he is a good sounding board, especially if I have a problem or am not sure how to deal with something, as often he's dealt with it or been in a similar situation. We often bounce ideas off each other which is nice of him.

More recently, I think Dr Marcus Hannon, although not a mentor but a really good colleague. I can pick the phone up to him anytime. He's now going through similar things to me at Aston Villa Football Club and hopefully I've helped him a little bit with my experiences that I have been through. It was always nice to have someone at the club day to day, so if I struggled with something, I was able to chat to that person about nutrition.

This can be a problem with the nutritionist industry; some individuals feel they can't speak to those in other disciplines, because it may seem like we don't know what we are doing. I think it's important that you get over that feeling and speak to other people in the club, or have mentors outside of the club who can pass on their nutritional knowledge and experiences.

We have a great group from Liverpool John Moores University, and I know the group are on hand at any time that I need them. It's a nice group of past and present PhD students who are honest and will give open and critical feedback.

I think doing my PhD has been one of the best things I have done, forming great friendships, and has been useful as a support network.

I'm a big supporter of the alumni that we've got from LJMU. So, as we look back from your dietetics studying to where you are now, is there a standout moment in your career that springs to mind?

Lloyd: Walking out of the tunnel during the Merseyside derby, I was standing outside on the pitch during the warmup with Jurgen Klopp (the Liverpool Football Club manager). I asked myself, "Is this real?" Many young children dream of being a professional footballer or an athlete. I was never going to make it, I was never good enough at any sport, in fact nowhere near good enough. But I'd always said from a young age that I would love to be involved in some way. I never thought I would get there, no one thought I'd get there, none of my friends or family. One of my mates was in the crowd as he is a Liverpool Football fan. He said to me "Mate, I can't believe it, you have literally got the best job in the world walking around Anfield doing the warmup during the derby!"

I think back and it is a cool "wow" moment. Obviously, there's a lot of history with Anfield and the size of the crowd, but also, I think when you're away from home it's sometimes even more special because it's an us versus them mentality and it brings you closer together as a group.

When you are the underdog and you have a smaller number of fans, it feels more special.

I love that! What's been the biggest challenge in your career to date?

Lloyd: I think one of the biggest challenges was believing in myself and that I deserved to be where I am. I think one of the things that I have struggled with frequently is impostor syndrome, whether it has been my PhD, or the applied roles. The feeling of "Am I good enough to work here or should I be working here?", that feeling of being found out. A lot of it comes back to this feeling. Sometimes I'd get paralysed by fear of my PhD and therefore didn't do any writing because of it.

I struggled in my first season at Everton Football Club. I went through a lot of lows, not many highs and part of that was the feeling of "Should I be here?", "What am I doing here?", "Am I the right person for the job?"

Hopefully this feeling drives me on to get better and to believe in myself more, but it's a struggle of mine.

At present, I'm not sure how I solve this. I will keep working hard and keep getting better, and eventually become more comfortable.

We all have elements of that at periods of our career; at certain times it's dialled up or dialled down. Moving forward, what characteristics do you think people need to work in the industry of performance nutrition?

Lloyd: You must be flexible; it's a volatile environment. I have been at Everton Football Club for four seasons now and I think I have worked with six managers and every manager wants things done differently. Every manager brings a different team of support staff around him, and players and staff around you are always changing. There are constant challenges, for example schedules are always changing. You've got to be flexible. If you are rigid in how you do things, you are just going to fail. You've got to be able to adapt, change to the environment and circumstances and what is required and demanded of you. In my role, I've gone from not travelling at all, to travelling to every game, to leading the whole thing, to having to work jointly with another nutritionist. There is this rollercoaster ride of things going on the whole time, so being flexible is key.

Naturally you have to work hard otherwise you won't survive in the industry. You have to put in a large number of hours, unsociable hours and weekends, especially if you do the travelling side of things in professional football. This gets even worse as you approach the Christmas period. If you enjoy your family life over the festive period, then this role is not going to be for you. For example, we have a game on the 19th December, the 23rd December, the 26th December, the 28th December. There won't be any days off. We will be in training Christmas Day. Boxing Day we are travelling and staying in a hotel for the whole day.

These roles have a shelf life. I do want some family time in the future, but right now I must be willing to sacrifice this in the short term if I want to be in the role. This is where I think people see the glorious side; they see you standing on the field kicking a ball around, but they don't see the side where you don't see your friends or family for weeks or months.

You've got to have the right mindset and to accept that sacrifices are needed in this industry. In summary, hard work, willing to sacrifice and be flexible are the main areas and of course willing to learn. This is the same for all top-end practitioner roles and in any field. If you ever think you've completed it or know everything, then you will become stuck very quickly.

What would be your biggest recommendation to your younger self or to aspiring students entering the industry now?

Lloyd: It is very different nowadays in some ways. When I started studying, Loughborough University was one of a handful who ran an MSc in Sports Nutrition. Nowadays, there are some great courses at Leeds Beckett University, LJMU and Chester University, to name a few. A lot more students are now qualifying and there are a lot of job opportunities which is fantastic, but it means that competition for each job is quite competitive.

Personally, I wish I had concentrated more in my first degree in sport science. I had moved away from home for the first time. I didn't know how to cook, didn't know how to wash clothes, didn't know how to look after myself and essentially just used the three years as a massive jolly-up. During the last year, I began to focus more and took it more seriously but for the first 18 months, I learnt little. I learnt life skills, but I learnt little academically. This pushed me back and meant I needed to do further studying. At the same time, it shaped who I am. For example, my weight gain is why I became interested in nutrition. Having said this, a small regret was not fully embracing what I could have learnt from great lecturers.

For other practitioners, find any opportunity and don't let your ego get in the way; don't say "I want to go straight into this club, with this team, or this sport". I started in rugby league and did not have a clue what the rules of the game were, as it was different from the rugby union rules that I already knew. But it was a great opportunity and I knew it would be good fun, so I went into it with all my effort. I learned all the rules and tactics behind it, went into the team meetings, and loved it. Even though it wasn't my sport, and I had no real interest in it, I soon developed a good fascination with it and I still watch it now and keep an eye on players I worked with. Take any opportunity you can even if it is not the sport you like, because you will still be building up skills that you will need for the future.

It's important to volunteer where you can, even if it's your local rugby club. You will be building up skills that you need for later and everyone wants practitioners who have experience. That's what you and I will be looking for when recruiting students. This may sound unfair, but you can go and volunteer somewhere. There's no excuse for it. Everyone's got a local rugby club or football club that hasn't got the funding to have a nutritionist, so knock on the door, find the right person to speak to and get the experience that you need.

When I volunteered at Saracens Rugby Club, I drove from Essex to Saracens. I did not earn anything and was spending approximately £150 a month on fuel, but it provided me with great experience. I had a full pre-season with the academy squad at Saracens Rugby Club and now a few of the players are in the England Rugby senior squad.

Lloyd: What you have described there is going above and beyond, isn't it? Some people laugh at you too, so for example, when I left the NHS, I was on a comfortable wage circa £20,000. Then the Manchester City Football Club role came up. I was living in Liverpool; I had just bought a house and so I couldn't move away. The wage at Manchester City Football Club was £15,000, so I took a £5,000 pay cut, plus I had to drive 80 miles each day. I was spending about £200–300 a month in petrol and only earning just over £1000 a month.

Friends asked me "What are you doing, you're 26 years old and earning £15,000?" However, for me it wasn't about the money. That's another thing I'd say about the sport nutrition industry. Don't join this industry if you're motivated by the money because it's not as well paid as you may think. You've got to love the job rather than think about massive salaries. Don't get me wrong, there are some big roles with big money but there is a lot of groundwork you need to do before you earn big numbers. As I said, I took a £5000 pay cut and even when I took the role at Everton Football

Club, again I accepted a pay cut. At the time Everton Football Club couldn't fund the role completely as it was a new role. If you're chasing money, then this is not the industry that you should be in, especially for the first 5–6 years of your career.

I was 30 years old when I finished my PhD and I was earning £14,500 tax free. I compare that to my old school friends who at 30 years old were earning approximately £90,000 in London.

Lloyd: That's the problem, you need to take that out of it. I was 26 years old and just started to work at Manchester City Football Club. Meanwhile my friends had already established a career and were earning good money. They were looking at me and thinking I am taking two steps back in my career. However, for me, it was a no-brainer, and I didn't think about the money. When I told people about the Manchester City Football Club role, they asked "What are you going to do?" I said, "I haven't even considered it, I'm definitely taking it. This is Manchester City Football Club Academy, working full time, it doesn't matter what the wage is." If I am honest, I would have done it for free for a year. It was a great opportunity. That was my view; there was no decision to make.

When I returned to university the second time to study dietetics, I was 22 years old. All my mates asked why I was going back to university and said I needed to get a career instead. They were beginning to earn disposable income and there I was at the end of university, 25 years old, still no job. However, for me it was well worth it and hopefully it has all paid off.

We spoke earlier about the number of courses that are available in our industry. However, do you think there is an area of sports nutrition that you didn't learn on your course, that's actually been really important for you, especially now you're working full time?

Lloyd: An area that I covered in my dietetics degree is behaviour change. How to do one-to-ones, how to extract information from people, how to coax people into changing behaviours and how to find out more information about that person. It's not about interviewing them but instead how to hold a conversation with them. It's a difficult skill to do well. To have a conversation with someone, to work out where you want the conversation to go and to think of a plan of attack. Combine this with knowing that you need to write your notes and finish in 10 minutes. There are many things on your mind and it's a skill that you need to learn. Some people are naturally better at it, of course.

I did a module on the dietetics degree although this wasn't enough; people didn't concentrate enough. Back then we did role play and it felt awkward. However, on reflection, it was very good. When I was in the NHS, we did a course on behaviour change and motivational interviewing. I found it useful and something that I have kept learning and progressing. There's a lot more behavioural research being published now which is great. Dr Dan Martin has done his PhD in behaviour change with jockeys and Dr Meghan Bentley has also studied behaviour change with her PhD. Although there's more research being published now in sports nutrition, we're definitely still way behind other industries in this area. If you look at the best MSc courses in the UK, there's not enough behaviour change content being taught. Even in sport science as a whole, even if you are not a nutritionist but a physiologist instead, the way you interact with athletes is so important.

You can know everything in the world but if people don't buy into you, they won't listen to you. Obviously, you need to know your knowledge, but these soft skills are so important. You need to know how to speak to someone to get your information across in the way you want it to land.

Another thing we are guilty of in this profession is an infographic. Many practitioners think they can put up an infographic and it ticks the box. It may look great, but it doesn't change behaviour. If you think how many times you have walked past infographics and not read the content. I was guilty of this at Everton Football Club. I put these amazing posters on the wall about food plates and models, fuel this and refuel that, have you recharged your battery, etc. I guarantee you, if you asked the players what words were on the posters, they couldn't tell you because the poster had become stale, almost like wallpaper. That's the biggest problem with these posters: they look at it once and then forget about it.

I think you're right, Lloyd. If you are going to put posters on the wall and you are going to have educational material designed, you should design it with the player. For example, educate them on how many carbohydrates they need on match day minus one, then ask them, what is it you want to see on this poster that will help remind you to increase your carbohydrates? Do you want to see a plate full of carbohydrates, or do you want to just see a huge "6g per kg body weight of carbohydrate" in big bold letters?

Lloyd: That's a great point. Speak to the player, ask them what their behavioural nudge needs to be to help them make better decisions. If you're going to put content on the wall, you should go digital because at least you can change it. I wanted to do this, but it was too expensive at the time for Everton Football Club. The problem with a static poster is you can't change it and it's stuck. We used a company who were very good who used magnetic posters. It allowed me to put stuff on top. This is something we could utilise more, but you will still be limited to what's on them already. If you go digital, it makes it easier to evolve your content. Additionally, as new players arrive, particularly national squads at England, if you have the ability to keep changing your nudges then you can evolve your education over time.

Where do you think the nutrition industry will be in five years' time?

Lloyd: That's a good question. I hope that as an industry we keep progressing. I think it's important we don't undervalue ourselves. A couple of years ago there was the danger of many people being consultants and us as nutritionists saying that being a consultant was enough. That's my big bugbear. I understand we need to take consultancy positions as people need to earn money and if the club only have budget to pay for three days' worth of work per week, then that's fine. However, think about how much impact you can really have on one day a week or one day every two weeks? For the people who take those roles, it's important they do a good job but also show how they could do an even better job, if they were in a full-time position.

Hopefully, we can keep pushing the industry in the right direction. I know I've tried to push the industry forward personally. When I was at Everton Football Club, I was asked what I wanted. I said that I would like a full-time nutritionist with the academy and a full-time nutritionist with the women, both supported by a PhD student. Unfortunately, the club weren't willing to fund that. Therefore, we decided to have Marcus (who was a PhD student at the time) doing three to four days a week and then the rest of the week focusing on his PhD. Now we've got someone there working 5–6 days a week.

At Everton Football Club, we achieved the outcome we were after by being strategic with the academic route. I still think we should have another nutritionist in the club; I think the role is too big for someone to do men's U23s down to U12s and the women side. Ideally, we need another practitioner at the club, and I'll be pushing for this in the next couple of years. I know Aston Villa Football Club now have Marcus and he has recruited a PhD student in the academy, so I think with good people in industry, who value it, we can begin to show the value of nutrition and what it can do.

We are still in danger of overvaluing it. In particular, the consultancy role can damage the reputation of the industry because clubs suddenly think wow, we are paying £X amount per day for this consultancy service and what is it they achieve? It can be difficult in nutrition to measure what you are doing apart from body composition assessments. I hope that clubs and teams begin to recruit full-time nutritionists, like how they've got full-time physiotherapists, performance analysts and sports scientists. For me nutrition is just 10 years, 20 years behind a lot of those roles as every club should also have a nutritionist. It is just as important but it's up to us to sell this message to those in charge of the money.

You're right, it is a discipline that we spend years studying, years becoming little experts. Yet it still falls on the lap of the fitness coach or sports scientist. Although more and more people are working full time in nutrition, there are still many jobs available. If you look at the 96 teams in the football divisions, maybe 40–50% have a nutritionist in the club. I am confident many of the lower teams do not have a nutritionist at all. There are still a large number of jobs to be had and I think you're right about the PhD model. We are biased to it because we've been through the PhD process, but for me if I was at a club, I would be recruiting a full-time nutritionist and funding a PhD student because you're getting the best of

both worlds. You have your own in-house research, potentially done with a full-time practitioner like I was at Warrington Wolves rugby and like Dr Marcus Hannon was with you at Everton Football Club.

Lloyd: You want succession at the club, you want continuity. For example, say I leave Everton Football Club tomorrow, the academy nutritionist would step up. He knows the area, he knows the system, he knows what we do, and then if you have a PhD model in there, they then take over the academy. Personally, I just see it as succession building. I'm not going to be in this role forever, so I want to make sure that when I do leave, it's in good hands and there's someone there that knows what they're doing and hopefully the club feel that they're ready to step up to the next level. From a club point of view, it makes sense, to make sure you have got consistency going forward. Hopefully, this is the way the industry develops.

Echoing what you have said, people reading this should know that 50% of clubs don't have a nutritionist in the Football League. With this in mind, there's a great opportunity for students straight away to reach out to those clubs and say, "I don't need paying at the moment, let me come into the club and I can show you what I can offer". Sometimes, it is as simple as that. You may get a no, but at some point, someone will welcome you in and open the door for you, giving you a small insight into it all and you can show them what you can do. Following this they may decide to pay you once a month as a retainer first and then suddenly you can quickly build and progress into more work.

If I was starting in this industry right now, that's where I'd be looking. I'd be reading this and thinking "Yeah, wow", more than half of football clubs in this country do not have nutritionists or any nutrition support. I will find the right person, share with them that I can offer my skills for free, send them my CV, and hopefully I will have the right qualifications and they don't mind me coming into the club for two or three days at first to see what they do and see if there is anything I can help them improve.

Is there a book that you've recently read, which has improved your practice or one that stands out?

Lloyd: I have not read a book recently, but I have read a recent case study by Dr Jose Areta, which was done over a five-year period on low energy availability. There's some really nice stuff coming out in that area. I think that's a huge area for me right now although we probably tried to jump the gun too quickly on it regarding the relative energy deficiency in sport on males and females. It's really interesting, however we are so far behind with the research and there are so many different nuances, particularly in females, so to get enough good research is going to take a long time.

What key principles do you try to follow every day?

Lloyd: Make your bed. A video I watched with a USA admiral said if you don't do anything else that day, at least make your bed. It's this notion of starting the day right, that results in better decisions that day. It may sound silly, but it certainly does start you off the right way. It's almost the official start of the day for me. Curtains open, make the bed, then I am ready for the day. It just gets you into a routine and signals to then get dressed. Especially during the lockdowns. That was a big learning curve for me. For example, if I lounge around in my PJs and I don't get up out of bed and don't open the curtains, then very quickly three or four hours have gone by. This then snowballs very quickly into the whole day wasted. In summary, I make the bed every day so I feel ready and then attack the day ahead.

Also having a few set goals of what I'm trying to achieve that day. If I'm going into work, I will have a task that I need to accomplish, but even personal tasks are important. It's a really nice feeling if you've got something to do and you can tick it off the list; it gives you a good buzz and it kind of actually makes you move onto the next task nice and quickly. With the PhD it highlighted areas that I need to improve. For example, procrastinating. I get paralysed by fear and if I see or look at a "to-do list" it scares me. Instead, I use a diary. I make notes in the diary of things that need doing but also at the end of the day write down everything I've done.

You realise how much you have completed daily by looking back at the jobs you have achieved. The problem with a "to-do list" is that you never finish them. You might have 16 things to do on your list; there are times when you might have 2 or 3 things left over when you get to the end of day and you feel like a failure because you haven't done everything you set out to do. This is when my mindset goes negative. Whereas, if you write everything down you've done that day, you can end the day on a positive note. You then go into the next day building on the previous day and so on.

I have previously used the "important/urgent matrix" which is pretty useful. In your opinion, what makes a successful performance nutritionist?

Lloyd: A person who can build rapport and change behaviour. Someone who can help your athlete to perform optimally as best as they can. We are such a small cog in such a big wheel; what we do is never going to win them something, but it could be detrimental if not done correctly, so you have to make sure that whatever that athlete is doing from a nutrition point of view, it is the best it can possibly be. They still might not win, but it doesn't mean they haven't done a good job; that's the most important thing to remember.

For a long time at Everton Football Club, I felt we were doing a really good job; you always try to improve things, but I thought we were 90% there at times. However, at certain times the team were playing really badly. Nutrition can only play a certain role in winning and it's important for those reading this book to remember that it's up to you to drive your own standards. It's up to you to make sure from a nutritional point of view, the players and the team are optimally fuelled and performing as best they can from your angle. You can't control a lot of the stuff on the outside, so don't get too high when it's good then get too low when it's low. Just concentrate on your role, and trying to change behaviours and make them the best they can be.

MY REFLECTIONS FROM LLOYD'S INTERVIEW

The first thing I would take from this interview is how Lloyd clearly followed the mantra of "jump and the net will catch you". Specifically, when Lloyd took the Warrington role, he was inexperienced, but importantly backed himself to do a great job and progress forward in his career.

Similarly, sometimes you have to go backwards in life to move forwards. Although it wasn't a difficult decision for Lloyd, not many practitioners would have had the courage to make a career move which resulted in earning less money. Again, this has only benefited Lloyd for the better as he has moved along his journey.

Advice from Lloyd about routines is a key tip that you can put into practice now. I have watched the video Lloyd references about the USA admiral and it is brilliant. I too make my bed every morning and get the curtains open to signal the start to a productive day.

For those who read this that want to get ahead of others in the industry, reading around the area of behaviour change is going to be key to your success as a nutritionist during your career.

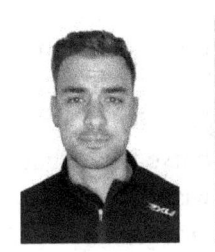

CHAPTER 3:
DR DANIEL MARTIN

Dan is a sport science and behaviour change expert undertaking a variety of roles, including Performance Nutritionist at Southampton Football Club, Performance Coach/Nutritionist at Haas Formula 1 Team, Lead Performance Nutritionist at the Professional Jockeys Association, Senior Performance Nutritionist at the English Institute of Sport (British Equestrian) and Post-Doctoral Researcher – Liverpool John Moores University.

He has worked as a performance nutritionist for eight years and studied his undergraduate degree in Sport and Exercise Science at Leeds Metropolitan, his Master's degree in Sport and Exercise Nutrition at Leeds Beckett University and PhD in Sports Nutrition, Education and Behaviour Change at LJMU. Dan was also awarded with the SENr Professor Clyde Williams OBE Award for Innovation in Sport and Exercise Nutrition Research and Education.

Dan and I first met when he joined LJMU to start his PhD in Sports Nutrition, Education and Behaviour Change. Both he and I had previously worked in rugby league and so over the last six years have shared many stories, over many beers, in Liverpool together. Dan was one of the LJMU PhD group and I have been fortunate enough to learn, develop and have fun alongside Dan during both of our studies at LJMU.

You can follow Dan on Twitter @nutritiondan

Could you give an introduction as to who you are and what your background is at the moment?

Dan: Most people know me for working in professional horse racing but that didn't come around until 2014. Before that, education wise, I had a very similar beginning to most of us in terms of an undergraduate degree in sport science. To be honest, initially I wanted to be a teacher or college lecturer. With this in mind, my next step in education was to study a Postgraduate Certificate in Education (PGCE) specialising in pedagogy and education which I completed at the University of Huddersfield.

Following this, I taught full time and started to do bits of nutrition on the side. I joined Leeds Beckett University to study a Master's degree in Sport and Exercise Nutrition. LJMU had not started their master's at that point, so I studied mine part time alongside working full time at Leeds Beckett University instead. At the end of my MSc, I had already built up some good momentum with some nutrition work, so I decided to take the plunge, quit my full-time teaching job and started a PhD at LJMU. This PhD was focused on jockey nutrition and education and behaviour change variables. This sums up the education background.

From the applied nutrition point of view, where I'm from in West Yorkshire, rugby league is the sport that you play growing up early on, therefore rugby league was the sport I always wanted to work in. I began working within the academy at Wakefield Trinity Rugby League, then my first senior team role was with Widnes Vikings Rugby League after you had moved over to Warrington Wolves Rugby League in 2015. From then, I've since transitioned into football. So, I had three seasons in first team rugby with Widnes Vikings and then went back to Wakefield Trinity for some time before working in football more recently with both Huddersfield Town Football Club and more recently Southampton United Football Club. As I said, most people probably know me for the work in the jockey world which started in 2014 and played a key role in me securing my PhD position in 2015. This was my first role getting paid what you could call secure money and working with full-time professional athletes. I've kept this role all the way through my career because the role is not a full-time position and it doesn't need to be right now.

You also work with motor sport, is that correct?

Dan: Yes, that's something quite new last season, working with Haas Formula 1 Team and my particular role is more with the team that sits around the two drivers. For example, the engineers or the mechanics. By definition these people may not be athletes, however if you understand the lifestyle and you understand the demands which are placed on them, then they are not normal mechanics or engineers. They are on the road travelling approximately 300 days per year; they travel through a lot of time zones. If they are attending back-to-back races, the mechanics will work 16-hour days for 5 or 6 days, have one day off, and then go again. With this in mind, general sport science and nutrition plays a big role in what they do, so although it's not an athletic population, like you may have with a football or rugby team, the principles of nutrition and sport science are the same. Although working with the drivers without doubt looks more desirable and that's what we all want to do, working with the support staff is a little bit more fulfilling because they don't get anywhere near the support or the money that the drivers get. As such, the impact you are making is probably, I guess, more impactful, than you might get with the driver.

So, your first full-time role in sport was at Widnes Vikings Rugby League?

Dan: I wouldn't actually say I've ever had a single full-time role within any of the clubs because my full-time role was always either as a teacher or followed by the PhD, and now as a post-doctoral researcher. On paper, the applied roles always came second to these roles. My first role within team sports at a senior level was at Widnes Viking Rugby, which you know as you were working there before me. To be honest, you left it in as good a place as anyone could leave it in, but the funds available in rugby league make it such a unique challenge compared to working in football. The budgets in football are considerably more than what they are in rugby which makes our job easier in some ways. It allows us to do a lot more stuff, although because in rugby you do not have a great budget, it does make you work a little bit smarter with the money you do have. I think that's always a good tool or skill to have in your armoury should you ever need to call on it again.

Definitely, I certainly experienced working under a tight budget at Widnes Vikings. Who were or are some of your biggest mentors so far and why have they been important for you?

Dan: Prior to nutrition, my first mentor was one of my colleagues in teaching and ironically, he was a professional rugby league player playing for Castleford Tigers before then signing for Widnes Vikings. I lived with him and now he is a head coach, but at the time he was teaching. I knew him as a teacher not as a rugby player and his teaching style was very different to other teachers that I observed during my teacher training. He controlled the room differently; the way he communicated, it was just better, a different level. As such, that was reflected in his teaching observations that he was graded on. I wanted to pick his brains, and in some ways I saw a lot of myself in him. He was one of the first mentors because he gave me the confidence to stand in front of a group of people, in a college where there were 20–25 learners in a room, and just be yourself. The aim was to develop and educate the students in a way that breaks the mould, rather than standing at the front and conforming to a teaching style that the other five or six people that I was observing at the time did. He did things differently and he put the onus very much on the students in a positive way. For example, he would teach for 90 minutes but only talk for 10 minutes; the other 80 minutes involved the students doing tasks, teaching themselves, teaching each other. It was very learning not teaching focused. I took the way that I worked as a teacher from him, into my nutrition roles. Even in those early roles when I was going to work in academy set-ups and doing work for free, I had my teaching approach in these roles, and it seemed to work well. I had the rapport with athletes; I felt I had the confidence to deliver the way I wanted to and not be a bit of an empty crisp packet stood up at the front of the room. Ironically, that style of teaching, he's taken into being a rugby league head coach and I've taken it into being a nutritionist. To be honest, I have never said it to him face to face, but he probably formed the foundation of how I operate as a teacher and as a nutritionist.

Moving into the nutrition world, you may say exactly the same but it's pretty obvious in Professor James Morton and Professor Graeme Close for similar reasons but also in unique ways. Graeme has got that gusto about him; when he is in a room, he owns it. He has a bit of fun but does it in a respectful way, and James has a work ethic and intensity which is just absolutely unrivalled and he's genuinely motivating to be around. I remember the first group meeting we had in 2015 when I first joined the PhD group, and he gave a speech. I thought it was a big motivational speech that he had prepared but it was just how he normally talks each day. James also owns the room and I think we have both been fortunate at Liverpool John Moores to have both of them as our supervisors, to look up to, to learn from and to have so many doors open for us. Additionally, by being part of LJMU, we've had the benefit of having their ears at any point during our journeys.

I know your career quite well just from being a good friend of yours, but what would be your standout moment in your career so far?

Dan: Unlike you, I have not won the League Leaders' Shield in rugby league, however some of the jockeys have been successful which is always rewarding and a nice feeling. To be honest, I'm a genuine sports fan and my biggest moments haven't necessarily been the team or the individuals winning something, but more so it has been the first experiences seeing what it's like behind the scenes.

I am a huge Formula 1 fan, and the goal has always been in one way or another to be involved in it or around it. The first time I got to see the car, it was like seeing an A-list celebrity. You know, you see them, and you can't help but stare and you think to yourself stop staring, but then you keep staring because you are not sure when you will see it again. I was in Singapore, and I walked through the back of the garage and the two cars were there and for me it was mental that the cars were just in front of me; it was electric! So, things like that I remember the most, even things like team talks. I have had the benefit of witnessing two or three different rugby head coaches deliver team talks. I think it's just fascinating the way the psychology and leadership styles are different. In particular, how rugby team talks are different to those in football and then you see two or three different managers deliver different team talks in football. For me, it's having that insight into the behind the scenes, that you never ever get as a normal sports fan sitting in the terraces. This is what gives me more fulfilment. You know, even if a team wins a trophy, you are obviously delighted, you can pose with a trophy, but it's those experiences that I remember most.

In a career sense, obviously attaining my PhD was a proud moment for me and more so for my parents as neither of them ever went to college let alone university, and then being recognised by the SENr committee and being awarded the Professor Clyde Williams OBE Award for Innovation in Sport and Exercise Nutrition Research and Education was great.

So, when you signed for Team Haas, was that a big moment for you in terms of F1 is the sport that you love and you are now the nutritionist for the team, so that must have been a nice day?

Dan: It's strange, I don't know if it's just me personally, but everything always seems like an anti-climax. I'm always then looking at what's next, and what's the next step forward. You sign the contract, and you think, yes this sounds great! It's the same when you submit your PhD... you do it and then you think "Oh, is that it?" I don't know what I expected but it is just over with far too quick. The moment the F1 job properly hit me was when I was first surrounded by the people and you see the car and you see the drivers; it's just an electric atmosphere around the place all the time. This was when the penny dropped. The first time when I actually got there, I guess I just didn't believe it. For me, until I got there and actually touched the car, I didn't fully believe it.

What do you think has been the most influential factor as to why you've been successful in your career to date?

Dan: One thing I've always done is work backwards from a destination. I've got friends that I started my undergraduate degree with and even did my master's course with and you look at where they are now. Not blowing smoke up either of our backsides, but I always knew what I wanted to do to some extent. Initially it was to teach but then I knew I wanted to work at the highest level of sport as a nutritionist; that was my passion. Once I knew this, I set my goals based on my destination. My goal was to work in both or either the Premier League or in Formula 1. If I'm honest, at the time working in F1 seemed like I was dreaming; it was like I wanted to go to the moon. This didn't stop me though; I set myself a destination and said right, that's the destination, so now I will work backwards from that. Regarding F1, I did my research and found a company called Hintsa who pretty much have F1 wrapped up in terms of work and support for companies and drivers. So, there was no way I could infiltrate F1 just on my own, so I looked at the people that worked there, what their qualifications were and what the entry requirements looked like. At the time, I was nowhere near it; I needed a PhD and a good body of experience behind me. So now the destination had been confirmed I knew I needed to study a PhD and get some experience. Therefore, for the next few years I got my head down, built up some experience, achieved the required qualifications and then I would be in a better position to apply to Hintsa and if successful, I would then be in F1.

I think because I have always had the destination in mind, I was always able to set out the path and the journey that I needed to take myself on. That's one thing I've always done, not just in sport, not just in work, just in everything really. If you can figure out where you want to be and how to get there, the path is quite easy to see, rather than just making it up as you go along.

There's nothing wrong with making it up for a while if you don't know your destination yet, but I think the sooner you have a goal or a destination that you have identified that you can work towards, the better.

I agree, this forms one of the presentations that I give to the John Moores University students every year. For example, how many people sign up for these degrees not knowing what it is they want to do? They just end up floating in the middle ground; they are in the washing machine just going round and round without any indication as to where they want to be or get to.

What's been the biggest challenge for you in your career to date so far?

Dan: The overriding one for me is finding a sensible balance. Early on in my career I said yes to a lot of things, got my head into everything and tried to figure some of the stuff out later down the line (i.e. how to manage it all). However, I've not let go of that mindset and I still say yes to lots of projects. For example, I have done this interview with you, although I am up to my eyeballs with different projects. Being involved in many projects is great, but I need to learn that I don't have to say yes to everything. This is the main thing that I am working on at the minute: learning how to have a better life balance. That's not necessarily saying for me to work less, but how to work smarter than I currently do.

At present, I've got an excellent mix of roles. I have my academic work and researching combined with work across a number of different sports with different cultures and subcultures. These all have different demands and at times that's fun and then other times it's really challenging. To go from a high-pressured environment or male-dominated environment and the next day going and working in equestrian, where it's completely different. These are my challenges; that's not to say everybody will have the same ones as me but for me it's all about finding that right balance.

I have reflected on this a lot. I'm not sure if it's part of the LJMU culture or way of working that we have all experienced. For example, I think of two individuals many of us would regard as mentors (i.e. Professors James Morton and Graeme Close), and we've seen how hard they work. Their workhorse mentality has been taught to many of us. Personally, I look up to both. I also look up to many of my colleagues and friends from LJMU. We had an amazing group that all pushed each other, and it breeds hard work. That's why a lot of alumni have progressed into some fantastic roles.

Many students at MSc and BSc level reach out to me on LinkedIn and ask for advice. A lot want the easy route all the time; people have to realise that simple hard work will help get you to the top.

Dan: Yeah, I couldn't agree any more!

What characteristics do people need to work in performance nutrition?

Dan: Work ethic is the big one. You want somebody that says yes and gives you confidence that they are going to do the job well. Someone who does the job with a smile on their face. They do the job with humility. Don't be one of those people, and we've all seen them, they do all the hard work until they get a tracksuit on. The tracksuit has their initials on and now they think they are big time! I always think to myself, what are you doing!? You have just undone all your good work!

There are fundamentals of any career path, be it sport or not. However, in sport I see a lot of people at the start of their journey with the fundamentals lacking. Sometimes it's cool to be uncool and not to be formal and I don't know why that is? For example, not wearing a tie to an interview or calling people "mate" too soon. Personally, people need to be tighter on those fundamentals, even if it does feel old school. Once you have settled in, you can then relax, but if you step over the boundaries too soon, you can't get that back. If you start too casual, you can't make it more formal because you have done the damage. Finally, someone with a strong work ethic and who is a good person. Somebody that is coachable, and wants to learn.

I agree, that's massive. Someone who is mouldable is ideal; you want someone that is willing to learn and be coached.

Looking back at your career, if a younger Daniel Martin or an aspiring student wanting to enter the industry asked you for your biggest recommendation, what would that be?

Dan: Do the things that we have mentioned. However, it is important to highlight that the industry is more congested than when we started.

Recently it has exploded with more courses and ultimately people graduating and seeking employment. Therefore, you've got to stand out, but for the right reasons. You don't have to do anything crazy, just do those fundamental things well and consistently. Put yourself under people's noses but be respectful in the way you do it. Say you'll do things and help out; sometimes it might be voluntarily, but do it well, with a smile on your face, and you'll be remembered for those things.

Stand out for being the person that asks questions and couldn't do enough for others and be polite while you do it. I think that's what's got me to where I am. Some of the guys from our PhD cohort are very clever cookies, and I'm not at the top of that particular intelligence tree, but I'm in the same mix and in the same circles work wise, because I do the fundamentals well. That doesn't make up for not doing your homework, not working hard and not doing the reading you need to do, but in the real world sometimes those qualities can be valued more than the PhD qualifications.

I agree and this leads into the next question. Are there any areas that you did not learn on the course that have been important for you now that you're working full time? We know how important the key principles of sport nutrition, physiology etc are. However, I think there are key areas that courses are missing, in terms of developing the individual in preparation for post qualification and ready for full-time employment. What courses do you think are missing?

Dan: Yeah, there are quite a few things. I appreciate universities can only fit so much into a master's degree programme, but even if there are selective modules that students can do in addition to the stock course, there are some basics that sport nutrition students don't get that everybody else seems to get. In particular, doctors and physiotherapists receive simple note-keeping guidance. My note-keeping system is probably OK but it's not perfect. I can't understand what doctors and physios write because they've been trained to keep notes in medical shorthand. I'm writing stories about the entire conversation that I had with someone, so I know what's going on, instead of using shorthand. I think we need to be taught better how to keep notes. Whether it's a client that you check in with every week, every couple of weeks or every month, or whether it's part of working in a multidisciplinary team. I'm not great at it; I'm only ok at it because I've had practice and had to do it. I've got better at it over the years but for the first 3–4 years after leaving the master's degree, I either wasn't keeping notes well or it wasn't very good practice. So that's one area.

A lot of us go into developing our own business. We don't all want to be an employee of a football club or a governing body. There's no support or training around how you develop your own business or limited company. For example, what's the best way to do it? It doesn't have to be a business and marketing degree but just a module on it would be very useful. At the moment, it's a lot of self-taught content that you do off your own back or spending money getting the advice of someone else. Media training is another area; not everyone will work in the media, but you and I are both on podcasts, we have both done a little bit of TV stuff or featuring in little documentaries etc, and I have frozen before! Even if it's just two or three sessions or three or four key points that you can take away from a master's degree. So, if you ever get asked to do an interview or be on TV, radio, podcast or write something for a newspaper, you at least have had a little bit of practice beforehand.

The biggest one out of them all is how to work and operate in the real world. We get taught the fundamentals on the course really well, but we don't necessarily get taught how to develop nutrition strategies from scratch. For the first 3–4 years I was a firefighter, going into the club or sport and on that particular day I was dealing with what was in front of me. For example, X wants a conversation, Y needs his skinfolds doing, Z wants a chat with you and then I would do that every time I went into the club. I would look back at the end of the season (thankfully I always asked myself because I'm quite a reflective person) and ask myself "Dan, show me how the club is in a better position going forward to next season, compared to when you arrived this season?"

If I couldn't answer this question, because I had put out hundreds of little fires, then I hadn't really made the club any better. Quite often, what I find is a club with no strategies in place. No one working directly with multidisciplinary teams, so when I now work within clubs, I try to develop a substantial nutrition strategy that aligns with the club's values, the goals that the MDT have set, all in the attempt to ensure the nutrition strategy is genuinely a part of the club. Additionally, I ensure that everything has documentation within the strategy policy, so if I was to leave tomorrow, the person taking over would know exactly what I've been doing and could theoretically run with it until they have a new nutritionist employed and then they could pick it up and carry on with it. We don't get trained to do this very well. We get trained to make people grow or make people thinner or adapt to training better, but we don't necessarily get taught how to develop the strategies that sit within MDTs.

I definitely resonate with the strategy area. In my previous roles, everything has to have a strategy with it and if it doesn't, and it doesn't feed into how we're going to allow a senior team to win competitions, then it doesn't get entertained.

Where do you think the future of nutrition will be in five years?

Dan: It depends on what we are talking about! In terms of glycogen or protein metabolism, probably not that far or not much further than what we already know! In terms of novel research areas, I think cannabidiol (CBD) will be a big area. There is a lot of funding available in this area at the moment. From a practitioner's point of view, I honestly believe it'll be the behaviour change and the implementation science. I've been lucky enough to study this early on in my PhD. My PhD was centred around this and there are only a couple of other people that are really doing research in this area at the moment within sport, so it's the vogue topic at the minute. Having said this, a lot of the conferences at the minute are interested in it and a lot of people are talking about it. Whether they are doing it right or wrong is a different question, but there are a lot of people talking about it. I think it's going to be a centre point of both research and practice for many years. I wouldn't be surprised if a lot more people are not just fighting fires that we're talking about, but they are actually developing interventions that are based on or grounded within behaviour change science. I think this will be a big area.

There are many people that will read this section who will resonate with that. Is there a book that you've read recently which has improved your practice?

Dan: *The Chimp Paradox* by Professor Steve Peters, it's not new, it's been around for a while. Professor James Morton has been telling me to read it for a while now. It helps you understand people differently. It certainly made me think a lot more before I speak or act, particularly if it's going to be in a negative way. Another book I'm reading at the minute is called *Dare to Lead* by Brené Brown. It's more of a leadership book, not that you have to be leader to read it, but it's about the power of vulnerability and getting people to change their behaviours in some ways. It's more about the psychology of trying to work with people.

Are there any key principles that you try to follow every day, that allow you to be successful?

Dan: One basic principle that comes from rugby, is something the All Blacks live and breathe by and that's "Don't be a d**k head". The other way of saying it is "just be a good person". At all levels, whether at work, at home, at leisure, whatever the scenario, be polite, be humble, do the right things. We all have a moral compass; make sure it's facing the right direction; don't antagonise unnecessarily. Apply your knowledge in the right way and you shouldn't be far off.

Finally, in your eyes, what makes a successful performance nutritionist?

Dan: Assuming that they are qualified, the best performance nutritionists are the ones that get on with and understand people best. They also happen to know a lot about nutrition as well.

MY REFLECTIONS FROM DANIEL'S INTERVIEW

I resonate closely with this interview, in particular the part where Daniel talks about being a good person. I have worked with many practitioners and support staff over the last seven years and the best relationships I have are with the people who are genuine and are a nice person... not a d**k head! Additionally, *The Chimp Paradox* is a book I am listening to now and it is brilliant.

Daniel clearly works in sport as he has a clear passion for being in this industry. Seeing the Formula 1 car for the first time is a nice reflection, but the key here was how important it was for Daniel to set the goal of working in Formula 1 and then working back from this. I often say to those I mentor that without a vision, you have no idea what your path should look like. Without a path you have no idea how to begin the journey.

Finally, it was nice to hear Daniel talk about his previous roles from teaching and how he now applies that into his day-to-day practice with the athletes he works with. I would ask you to reflect on any of your previous roles and how the skills you have learnt can be transferred into performance nutrition. For example, you may have previous experience working in hospitality where communication and timing skills are huge. Similar skills are key when working with hotels under time restrictions to arrange and confirm the menu you need providing for your team.

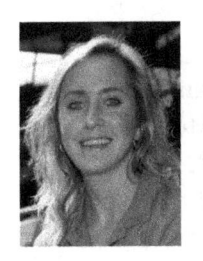

CHAPTER 4:
HANNAH SHERIDAN

Hannah has spent the last six years working at the elite level of sports nutrition and currently works as the Lead Sports Nutritionist at Tottenham Hotspur Football Club. Her undergraduate degree was in Sport and Exercise Science from the University of Birmingham. Following the undergraduate degree, Hannah then progressed on to a Master's degree in Sports Nutrition from the University of Stirling.

Hannah and I first met at the International Sport and Exercise Nutrition Conference in December of 2017 which is hosted in Newcastle every year. It is a great conference and one that all young practitioners should be attending. Hannah and I had some great discussions about what we were both studying and where we were working at the time and since then have always stayed in touch and shared experiences and challenges with each other.

You can follow Hannah on Twitter @HSperfnutrition

Could you just give a brief introduction as to who you are and what your background is?

Hannah: I'm currently the Lead Sports Nutritionist at Tottenham Hotspur Football Club, where I work with the first team. We've recently employed an academy nutritionist to take some work out of my hands.

To start with, I went to the University of Birmingham and studied my undergraduate degree in Sport and Exercise Science. I used to be an athlete myself, I did a lot of sports, but in particular I did a lot of athletics. Athletics at Birmingham was really good; the team was good, and the coach was one of the best in the country. The sport science undergraduate degree at Birmingham was also one of the best. I went there for three years and in my final year I specialised in sports nutrition.

Within the course, there were two study options: either a psychology focus or a science focus, including modules such as biochemistry and physiology. It was the latter which interested me and I knew if I studied the correct modules it allowed you to do the sports nutrition module. I loved this module. There was a practical element to it and that stemmed from the lecturers and the researchers that were there at the university. These included academics like Professors Kevin Tipton, Asker Jeukendrup and Dr Oliver Witard.

Asker, in particular, had a great background in the applied side as well as research which was attractive. I was lucky enough to have him as my dissertation tutor and so I learned from him in the lab but also outside of that as well. Understanding what he was doing outside of university was great and I just thought, this is what I want to do.

I found my final year difficult, quite stressful, so after I finished my undergraduate degree, I took a break. I was certain that I was going to study sports nutrition, but I didn't want to go straight into studying a master's. I got a job working for Dame Kelly Holmes.

Kelly ran a female athlete initiative for the top female athletes in the country at teenage age. Her aim was to keep them in the sport and competing at this age. Kelly used her team of practitioners that helped her through her own Olympic cycles. For example, there was a sports nutritionist, a sports doctor, a sports physiotherapist and I was the coordinator of the events. Whilst doing this, I was exposed to the elite environment. On reflection, because I hadn't made it to the elite level myself as an athlete, I decided that's where I wanted to work as a member of staff.

It wasn't the general population or clinical work in a hospital that excited me, it was the sport side. I did that job for about a year, and then I was ready to carry on my studies. I decided to do the International Olympic Committee (IOC) Sports Nutrition diploma. This course was similar to a part-time graduate course. I knew that one of the things that would help me be successful in the world of sports nutrition was getting work experience, and this would make me stand out from the hundreds of other candidates who were also studying.

So, alongside studying the diploma, I started working in the Women's Super League for Watford Football Club. I worked with Watford for two seasons, whilst balancing paid roles to help fund my course and general living in London. At the same time, I had a part-time job working in a school as a teaching assistant with special needs children. This job was challenging, and you had to adapt your ways of working with the children. I learnt many skills from this role that helped me to become a better practitioner. They helped me work with a diverse range of athletes and adapt my communication to different learning styles.

Overall, I was balancing all three roles (paid work, voluntary experience and my studies), but I loved it and knew 100% this was what I wanted to do. I carried on gaining experience and also worked with the local diving squad, doing workshops for parents and accumulating different experiences with different sports.

Once I'd finished the IOC diploma in 2014, I travelled north to the University of Stirling, Scotland and completed my master's conversion with Professor Stuart Galloway. I graduated from my master's a year later and then went into full-time work in the applied field.

I was lucky. It was almost perfect timing to be honest. At the time I was still studying in Stirling and I was gaining work experience with the Scottish Institute of Sport. A job at the high-performance centre in Birmingham was available and I took the role. It was with various elite athletes, for example GB hockey players, GB swimmers, GB athletics and individual athletes who attended the high-performance centre. It was client based and I loved that role, working with the psychologists, physiotherapists and doctors. I learnt a lot and I think one of the best bits of that job was that it was so varied. I learnt a lot about the demands of all different sports, working with loads of coaches, and a variety of athletes of different ages.

I was there for nearly three years and then the role at Tottenham Hotspur Football Club (Spurs) was available which is located 20 minutes from where I grew up. It was time for me to go back home. Therefore, in 2017 I moved back to North London and started the role at Spurs as a sports nutritionist with the first team. At the start of this role, I worked alongside another sports nutritionist, Maria Porter, who had come over from Barcelona, and then Dr Sophie Killer.

Amazing. Everyone's got a journey and it is nice to hear yours. I think there are a lot of students who graduate and think they can do an undergraduate degree, they can do a master's degree and then all of a sudden, it's like "Oh yeah, I've got a job".

Hannah: 100%. That's why I would say everyone's journey is different and you've got to follow what's right for you. Above all you've got to love it and also just go the extra mile to stand out from the rest of them. There are many candidates now, and maybe we were lucky at the time when we graduated as it wasn't quite as popular, even though it seemed so at the time. The popularity of sports nutrition courses has exploded.

I agree! When you went from Birmingham to Spurs, was the job available? When you put your application in, were you confident that you were going to be successful?

Hannah: It was weird how the job came around. I was approached about it. One of the sports scientists had spoken to other practitioners and asked if they would recommend anyone. I hadn't actually seen the role advertised and I knew I had to go for it. At the time, I hadn't worked in full-time football, but I had worked with individual footballers so I had a good understanding of the game and the demands of the game.

I was required to do a presentation for my initial interview. My first interview involved presenting to the manager, assistant manager, head of sport science and head of medical. I presented the nutrition frameworks that I use and what sort of things I would do initially if I was to get the job. There hadn't been a full-time role before at Spurs which was interesting. They only had someone in once every two weeks so there weren't too many strategies in place. I presented my framework and philosophy, and it seemed to go well in the interview. I was confident I was in a good place. I then had a one-to-one interview with lots of questions and it was weeks till I found out if I had been successful or not. It was classic football; nothing happened for a while. I started doubting myself. I knew they'd flown people over from America and various places to be interviewed. When I found out I was successful, I was absolutely buzzing.

Well, many congratulations; it is amazing to see good friends doing well in the industry.

So, through that journey and through your path so far, who would you say some of your biggest mentors have been in your life and why are they important for you?

Hannah: From an early age my personality traits have been developed from my parents. They always taught me that failure would only help you and you could always come back from failure. I was never the cleverest kid and I had to work hard. My parents never pushed me, but they supported me a lot and so I would say my parents had a big influence on me growing up. Before the interview with Tottenham Hotspurs, I attended lots of other interviews and failed. I had to pick myself back up from what was a tough situation, but my parents were always there for me and believed I could come back from those failures and setbacks.

From more of an academic point of view, I would say Oliver Witard during the period of time when I was studying at Stirling University. I knew Oliver from Birmingham University, and I was moving pretty far away from home (seven-hour car journey) and didn't know anyone. Oliver was a familiar face and he had previously studied at Birmingham University, completed his PhD, and so he helped me.

In particular, he helped with the scientific writing which progressively became more difficult for me. I enjoy the applied side of nutrition, but the scientific writing doesn't come naturally to me. He was a really good support whilst at Stirling University. Oliver also helped me settle into the local area which ultimately led to me starting a full-time applied role. I would say he's been a great mentor and I know I could pick up the phone to him if I needed some advice or anything like that. He's also done some applied roles and is absolutely brilliant in the research field.

Many of the people I have interviewed have said similar about being able to embrace lessons. A failure is only a failure if you don't learn from it, therefore it becomes a lesson. I completely agree with you.

What is a standout moment for you in your career to date?

Hannah: I'm sure you're thinking it will be the Champions League Final, but for me it would be the game that got us there. The Champions League Final was heartbreaking actually. Playing Ajax Football Club away was our semi-final. It was the second leg, and we were 1–0 behind on aggregate when we started the game. They beat us 0–1 at home. We went to their stadium and the first half was disastrous. I remember walking in at half-time and thinking, well this is done; we had to score three goals in the second half to get through and we'd been playing terribly. There was a lot of fighting talk in the dressing room, but I don't think it even entered my head that we would score three goals, to the point where I'd stayed in the changing room for most of the second half because I was thinking to myself, the food after the game needs to be perfect, because otherwise there could be food all over the place at this rate!

I was in the changing room and we scored the first goal, which gave me hope. I remember our kit man said that whatever he predicted the score to be, it would be. He said, "Hannah, we're going to get two more goals." I was thinking, "Don't be ridiculous, that is never going to happen." Sure enough, they scored two more goals, and we won the game. Honestly, it was unbelievable.

I was by the side of the pitch, next to the bench after the third goal. There were 30 seconds left in the game and I was holding onto the doctor's hand. It was a big adrenaline rush to come from such a low to such a high. Against all odds, to come from behind, was crazy.

The Champions League run of games was special. We played Manchester City Football Club away a couple of weeks before that which was a crazy game too. Altogether, as a member of staff, you're so invested in the whole process, in every game, especially the Champions League! That was really special for me.

There are a number of things that you mentioned here. The first area I want to revisit is how in the depths of the Champions League semi-final, the first thing you're thinking about is how good the food needs to be! I remember watching that game and I remember seeing you on the pitch after; there is an amazing picture of you with the manager and I think when we all look back at our careers, it's moments like this, where you can say, "I was there for that night", and not only physically there, but in that emotional moment there was a brilliant connection between staff and players.

Hannah: Yeah, I would definitely say that I had a good connection between the staff, coaches and the players. At that moment, it was like there were no rules. You think back to it now and think that wasn't normal from a professional point of view; you wouldn't just run on the pitch when we score a goal in general, but for this game everything went out the window.

We couldn't even process that there were cameras around or anything; it didn't even enter our minds. Emotions were all over the place.

What do you think has been the most influential factor as to why you have been successful to date?

Hannah: In my own sporting career, I had to learn to be determined and dedicated. I've then been able to translate that into my professional career. As we've said, sports nutrition is hard to get into and you've got to be resilient and you've got to be dedicated, determined and keep going. There will be setbacks and it's not just as simple as graduating from university and applying for a job anymore; there's so much more to it than just that.

I'd say being successful comes from my underlying personality traits that have stemmed from my sporting background. I knew I wasn't naturally as talented as some of the other athletes I used to train with, however I stood out because I was so determined to progress, be the best and never give up. In summary, I'd probably say determination and resilience have been essential.

What's been the biggest challenge of your career to date?

Hannah: The transition from Olympic sport into full-time football. I wasn't in a centralised environment when I was at the high-performance centre in Birmingham and usually had weekends off. I think we could agree, football players are just completely different athletes to Olympic athletes. It probably stems from the culture that is created in professional football nowadays, and maybe the money has something to do with this as well. Football has a lot of luxuries compared to other professional sports.

On one side, you've got Olympic athletes, that will do anything you tell them to do, whereas football is a little different. There is a little bit of "I'm here, I'm at the top of my game, why should I do these things you are telling me to do?"

So, for me this was a tough challenge: the change in environment, and also the complete change in lifestyle. Working weekends can be tough all season long and time off over Christmas doesn't really exist in football. This was a big shock to me; I had to do a lot of adapting. If I am honest with you, I spent some time working out if this was what I really wanted to do, and over time I have grown to love it.

You build relationships with coaches and players, and I think you begin to learn a bit more about the different personalities in the team and how you can motivate them to be better. You start learning more about the culture of the club and you get to adapt to that. If you can deal with how different it can be sometimes and you like it and you enjoy it, you'll adapt to that lifestyle. In summary, the actual lifestyle change is probably the biggest challenge in my career so far.

We have both worked in football. Do you think the success of the gold standard nutrition practices that we would all like to do with our athletes is hampered by the culture of the sport, or do you think it's limited by ability of the practitioner to actually coach the individual player?

Hannah: Absolutely. When I first went into the club for the first two seasons, there were players that I thought I would never be able to change in terms of nutrition habits. To try to get any player, well quite a high proportion of them, to engage in things, was hard. They didn't have much interest and then gradually as you start doing more individual work with them you get to know them better. Some of the real challenging players have taken me three seasons to get through to and it might be just one little conversation and you see them engage in something you've been pushing for three seasons. You think to yourself, wow, it's worked; I've finally worked out how to motivate them or know what makes them tick.

It's a bit of a mix. The culture of football doesn't help, but equally, if you know you're a person that can build relationships, and you are personable and flexible in your style of working, you can have good successes. One of the things that Craig and I are really proud of this season is the outcome of the pre-season workshops we delivered.

We did small group workshops to educate key players about supplements, such as beta-alanine, which players normally do not take consistently well. I know it may sound silly but normally after a week or so there will be three of them consuming it. Out of the squad of 26 this season, only five players are not consuming it. The only thing that we've done differently is to spend time speaking with them about the benefits for their performance, rather than just putting up an infographic or putting it in their shakes and hoping they take it.

The coaches' support of the group workshops was really helpful. We put some of the younger players with the senior players and it worked well together. It was an opportunity to ask lots of questions. I told them, everything is your choice, we're not forcing you to do this, but I'm telling you this is why it's important for you and this is how it can affect your performance. I was trying to get across that I am not standing here wasting my time; I wouldn't promote something that doesn't work. We showed them the research and we made it player friendly.

The buy-in this season has been brilliant. We haven't had any complaints and for Craig and me, it was an eye-opening moment. In four football seasons, I have never had so many of them compliant with this strategy. With education and time, you can definitely get the outcome you are after. This season proved it for me.

What characteristics do you think people need to work in performance nutrition?

Hannah: Definitely passion. This will then have a knock-on effect on your determination. If you love what you do then you're going to keep working hard for it and you won't necessarily see it as work.

I think resilience is big. There are going to be setbacks and you need to motivate yourself to come back from those. I think you need to be personable and have really good communication skills because, like I've explained, you've got to adapt the way you work with different players. You've got to understand how different athletes or players are motivated, what makes them tick. To do that, you've got to have good communication skills and be aware of different personalities. Also, it's good if you can be quite flexible in elite sport. It's not Monday to Friday 9–5. A lot of the time it's unsociable hours and if you want to work at the top level then you've got to be flexible and work around those challenges.

In summary, passion, determination, resilience, personable, good communication skills and then flexibility.

What would be your biggest recommendation to your younger self or to aspiring students entering the industry now?

Hannah: My younger self, I think I would say be better at reflective practice. It's not a human instinct to critique yourself and look at what you're bad at. However, I think in the last five years, more master's courses are teaching modules on reflection and there's a lot of reflective practice that you have to complete and submit when you do the Sport and Exercise Nutrition Register (SENr).

I completed my insights profile about five years ago and it produced five pages that explained me word for word. I knew these things. I knew what my weaknesses were, but I'd never addressed them. When I read them, I thought to myself, now it's time to try and improve on some of these. For example, one of mine was attention to detail. I don't enjoy monotonous tasks with data. I hate Excel, but I knew that for my work it would make me a better practitioner. Reviewing results and trends is needed sometimes and to start reflective practice and to look at your weaknesses, teach yourself what they may be, this would have been really valuable for me.

For practitioners starting, or in the industry now, I would say follow your own path. Don't look at what everyone else is doing. You might see people finishing undergraduate degrees and going into a PhD, but actually, if that's not what excites you, don't do it. It's not a route for everyone. Loads of people have done great work going into a PhD and then into the applied field, then others, like myself, haven't gone down the research side so much yet. That's because at the time, that wasn't right for me. I completed the International Olympic Committee Diploma and then my master's conversion. This isn't the most popular route of study, but it doesn't mean it was the wrong one. Go with what you feel is right at the time as you'll get the most out of it.

It's an important point. There are many different options or paths to take and you have to find the right option for you. Are there any areas that you didn't learn on the course that you think would have been important for you now that you are working full time? You mentioned the reflective practice. I agree with you, that's an important area that we don't get taught on, but is there anything else that stands out for you?

Hannah: It's such a new and emerging area, but behaviour change. A lot of the work I do, the nutrition physiology side and our guidelines and recommendations, are pretty solid now, but it's actually working out what are the barriers and enablers for different players so that we can get them to engage in these strategies. This is something we're not taught, but it's good to see it's an emerging area of research at the moment. Incorporating behaviour change into a master's course or even an undergraduate degree would be valuable. Everyone can learn what protein and carbohydrate guidelines are for football. These guidelines are not changing massively anytime soon, but an understanding of why that player is not doing what you may have asked or how can you get them to do it better – this is where you're going to find the most value and it's important. I definitely think behaviour change would be useful for students to study on courses at the moment.

Where do you think the future of nutrition will be in five years' time?

Hannah: There's a big focus on individualising and personalising nutrition plans and strategies for various athletes. The involvement of nutrigenomics is interesting. Looking at genetics and how that might influence how athletes metabolise, excrete or absorb a certain nutrition is something that is exciting. A key finding from this sort of knowledge could be around caffeine guidelines for example. Loads of players take caffeine before a game, but we don't actually know if this is detrimental to one player but really useful to another based on their genetics. I think, in the next five years, this line of work will carry on evolving. Hopefully there will be a simple way of looking at it for individual athletes.

I read a paper the other day that looked at the energetic loss in faecal. It looked at how much energy individuals absorbed from the food that they were consuming, but also how much energy they lost because their gut wasn't absorbing it and therefore, they were losing energy in their poo. I think it was in the region of a 150kcal swing in some of the energy that people absorbed, comparing one person to another.

Is there a book you've recently read which has improved your practice?

Hannah: Lockdown has actually been a great time for me to read; I don't often get time to do it. I read a book called *The Culture Code* by Daniel Coyle. It's not just about successful sports teams but also successful businesses. It looks at companies like Google and Pixar and the United States Navy SEALs.

It's really interesting. They analyse why these businesses and teams have been so successful. You read it and think to yourself that if we could implement that in our team that would make it a better place to work. Simple things, like making sure people feel like they belong, creating safety and creating trust through sharing your vulnerabilities. A lot of things you may think you currently do really badly and other things you might think you do quite well. For me, to be able to go back into work and share those ideas amongst people is important. One thing with football is it doesn't always create a feeling of safety. We know it can be such a cut-throat environment. If we can create a better environment, we would probably be even more successful. That was a great book, nothing to do with nutrition, but more about creating a successful environment.

Are there any key principles that you try to follow every day?

Hannah: Yes, always give 100%. There are always menial tasks that you don't like doing but you know the result of the task is bigger than the actual task. For example, making up the recovery shakes, you've got all these individual ingredients you put in the shake. You could easily think, I can't be bothered. However, you know the impact it's going to have if you do that one task correctly every day. It is huge.

In general, I would say being a good person; try to help someone out each day. Lastly, I would say, especially in nutrition, stick to what you believe in. If you know someone is about to challenge you that's fine; everyone's got an opinion on food, and if you know your opinion is right, then you should justify it. Obviously choose your moments. A good example may be if a coach is telling me they think a player is fat, when actually they're not fat. They may have put on 2kg of muscle mass because they have been doing extra work in the gym. You could cause problems for the player by agreeing with the coach and allowing them to think he was "fat". Therefore, you need to explain it in the right way to the coach and justify it. Essentially make sure that you stick to your values as this is important.

In your eyes, what makes a successful performance nutritionist?

Hannah: Being passionate, driven, a good communicator and determined. In nutrition, your communication skills are just as important because being successful in this role is based on how well you can communicate something and motivate your athletes to change their behaviour. You really have to be passionate about food because it is something that comes naturally to everybody every single day i.e. eating food. Therefore, it is your task to make it exciting. You need to love your work, food and nutrition and be imaginative with it as well. You have to create performance foods or sports foods. They might not always taste great when they're just in powder form but how could you incorporate this into a snack or a meal and get the players and athletes to buy into it?

MY REFLECTIONS FROM HANNAH'S INTERVIEW

Isn't it interesting again to hear another successful practitioner talk about how her journey has been so unique? This highlights how there really is no direct blueprint as to how to get that first job in the industry.

One thing that stands out here for me, however, is how Hannah has worked hard from the beginning. Whether this was her as a younger athlete, or the fact that she was willing to put her hand up and gain experience with the Dame Kelly Holmes Trust, it was all about gaining the front-facing experience.

Hannah has also been smart in her approach to her applied work. Learning lessons from previous roles but also times where she may have done something wrong, but then reflected on that moment and learnt from it.

Being a good person and willing to help others again has popped up, which is similar to what Daniel Martin said in the previous chapter. Finally, a big standout point that Hannah states, and one that resonates with me strongly right now, is that you have to have passion for your role. If you do not have passion, you are not going to enjoy what you do. There is a fantastic podcast by Eddie Hearn, from Matchroom Sport, called "No Passion, No Point" and this refers to exactly the point Hannah is making here.

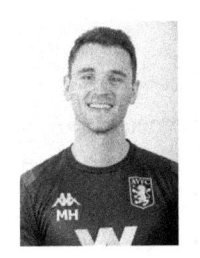

CHAPTER 5:
DR MARCUS HANNON

Marcus has been practising as a performance nutritionist for the last six years, having previously worked as a nutritionist at Everton Football Club within the academy before his current role as Head of Nutrition at Aston Villa Football Club. His undergraduate degree in Nutrition and Sports and Exercise Science was from Oxford Brookes University. He then went on to study his Master's degree in Sports Nutrition before recently completing his PhD in Applied Physiology and Sports Nutrition, both from Liverpool John Moores University.

Marcus and I met at the International Sport and Exercise Nutrition Conference (ISENC) in Newcastle in 2014 and since then have remained very good friends. We often call each other to bounce ideas off one another and share experiences and lessons.

You can follow Marcus on Twitter @marcushannon92

We know each other well from our time studying together in Liverpool. Could you give an introduction into yourself and your background, where you've come from and what you are currently doing?

Marcus: I am originally from sunny Belfast, Northern Ireland. I grew up and did all my school years there. After school and college, I spent a year abroad in Australia and was a sports coach in a school. After that my higher education career started like most of us. I studied my undergraduate degree at Oxford Brookes University (OBU). The course was a combined honours degree in sport science and nutrition, and it was brilliant. At the time (2013–2016), there were only a couple of courses in the UK offering the two together. I always knew that I wanted to study sport nutrition. OBU was my second choice; my first choice was with Glasgow University to do the same degree, however I didn't get the grades to attend Glasgow. I don't know if the course is still running at OBU, but it was this course which allowed me to study the core nutrition modules and the core sport science modules together as one. As you know, a lot of students end up studying modules that they may not want to, just to make up content.

I enjoyed a lot of my undergraduate degree because I was able to study what I wanted to. In my last year, I contacted the local sports team which was Oxford United Football Club who were playing in League Two at the time. Although they were a professional football club, at the time they were right at the bottom of the league. I contacted Alistair Lane, who was the head of sport science, and he invited me in to meet him, which I did. We had a bit of a chat and I asked him if there was any chance I could come into the club to gain some experience. He said no problem and during that last year, I attended the club on average once a week. It was more shadowing than anything else to be honest, but I knew it was going to help me out in the future. I helped where I could, collecting balls, cones, water bottles, all those little jobs. As the year progressed, they asked me to do a little bit more. For example, making the sports drinks, making up supplements, performing hydration tests. Oxford Football Club was really my first exposure to professional sport and although it was good, it wasn't very professional. I laugh now but the manager's office and the gym were in a little portakabin; the pitches were fields in the local area. Irrespective of this, it was a great experience.

After OBU, I moved back home to Belfast to save up some more money ready for a master's degree. During this time, an opportunity arose to do some strength and conditioning work with Ulster Rugby within their academy. Although I was saving up and wanted to study sport nutrition, there were no opportunities or openings at the time in that space. To be honest, I thought to myself, look there's an opportunity to do some strength and conditioning here, I was interested in it and also this experience would expose me to more professional sport.

At the time, Ulster Rugby delivered strength and conditioning services to local schools. I led this programme for a couple of the schools and was also involved in their Academy Pathway programme, which was with the age-grade athletes. I coached and assisted the current strength and conditioning coaches. I did this for a year whilst working in a bar to save up for my master's. I think that's about the time I met you at ISENC. This was back in December 2014 in Newcastle. At this time, I had the intention of doing my MSc and postgraduate degree in sport nutrition at University of Ulster in Belfast to save a few pounds. However, over the course of this year I thought this probably isn't the best master's course that is on offer. I had thought about Loughborough University and LJMU. Then after meeting you and some of your colleagues at ISENC, it was obvious that LJMU was the place to be and that's where I wanted to go.

I moved over to Liverpool and studied my Master's in Sport Nutrition at LJMU. This was an unbelievable year, learning from some of the best in the industry and getting involved in research projects. During this year, there was a placement at Wasps Rugby Club based in London. Me and another guy, Richard Kelly, used to travel down to London every two weeks for two days at a time to do our placement with the team. This allowed me to gather even more exposure to professional sports but this time it was solely nutrition which was great. Once I finished up my master's and the placement, an opportunity arose to do an applied PhD in collaboration with Everton Football Club. I spent just over three years at Everton Football Club leading on the academy nutrition with a great team of nutritionists. This was a brilliant learning experience for me and alongside the day-to-day work, I collected my PhD data and research. During this time, I also spent a year with Northampton Saints Rugby Union senior squad and in January 2020, I joined Aston Villa Football Club as Head of Nutrition.

Your first exposure to nutrition was with Oxford United Football Club?

Marcus: Correct. I was performing hydration testing and making up supplements and sports drinks. Back then I didn't really know what, why or when to do certain things. I had an idea, but I didn't know about the finer details. I would speak to players about nutrition but again, I wasn't qualified to do this properly at that stage. It was only when I did the master's that I started to learn about things in more detail and in greater depth. My placement in the real world was probably the first experience of providing specific advice to individuals and athletes.

As you think about your career so far, who were, or who are some of your biggest mentors in your life, and why have they been important for you?

Marcus: First and foremost, my mum and dad. They exposed me to success. They were both successful in their careers and the first thing that they showed me is work ethic. They used to work very hard. My dad is retired now, and my mum is winding down, but I know they worked very hard throughout their careers. They've mentored me and continue to mentor me now – I speak to them most days!

From a professional point of view and from a career point of view, I had a great lecturer called Dr Charlie Simpson from OBU who taught me on the specific sport nutrition module. Charlie is a fantastic teacher; I thoroughly enjoyed his classes. I always had a passion for sport nutrition, but Charlie really solidified and ignited that passion even further.

I did my undergraduate placement with Dr John Jakeman – he was brilliant and provided fantastic advice and mentorship. Then when I came to LJMU, Professors James Morton and Graeme Close have been outstanding. It was due to these two that I studied at LJMU, because of who they are, what they did and what teams they were involved in, and their sort of status within the sport nutrition world. They are and continue to be my two most important mentors.

What would be a standout moment in your career to date?

Marcus: It's interesting as before we started the conversation together, I was saying how the goalposts (goals and ambitions) always move and always change. When you get your undergraduate degree you tick that box, then you go into your master's and you tick that box, and then you go on to get your PhD. You get to the day where you have your viva and you're successful in it; it's a brilliant day. I don't know if they are milestones along the way, however there are stages that I have been proud of from an academic point of view. One thing that does stand out was presenting some of my research at the Union of European Football Associations (UEFA) headquarters. That was a real highlight. To be invited out to speak to the Sports Science and Medicine Research Board at UEFA in Switzerland was special and I received positive feedback. Getting offered a job as Head of Nutrition at Aston Villa Football Club was also special. Five or six years ago I wouldn't have thought I'd be in the position I am in now. It's nice and I'm very proud.

Is there a game since you've been at Aston Villa Football Club that is memorable?

Marcus: We went to Wembley Stadium last season as we managed to reach the Carabao Cup Final. We were narrowly beaten by Manchester City Football Club 2–1. Although we were beaten, that was a special day. We also beat Liverpool Football Club earlier this season 7–2 who were the current Premier League Champions. That was a special night. We've been to Arsenal Football Club and beat them 3–0 this season as well. It's been great and hopefully there are many more of those nights to come as well.

What do you think has been the most influential factor as to why you've been successful to date? What is it Marcus has that other people might not have?

Marcus: I wouldn't say I have anything that others don't. However, one thing that myself and you certainly have, and others who've come through the LJMU pathway on the PhD model, is just a hard work ethic. To be able to complete an applied PhD where you're in a club full time and working a full-time job can be hard at times. At Everton Football Club I oversaw the academy nutrition; we had 115 players all of whom have parents or host parents and guardians that need educating. They all want some time with you; it's such a big job to try and do well. Personally, clubs should have two or three nutritionists within an academy. I was doing that and then trying to do my PhD, and it was an enormous task, but for the three and a half years that's what I did. I just got on with it. I worked pretty much every weekend and worked 12–14-hour days. You have got to just put the graft in. You don't have to be the smartest person in the room, but if you can work hard, you will go far in your career.

One thing I've done consistently well through my career is networking. For example, I met you way back in 2014 at ISENC. I saw that conference online and it was £300. I didn't know anyone going and it was in Newcastle; I was in Belfast at the time. I had never gone to conferences before and I remember thinking, can I afford that? I thought sod it, so I paid it, booked my flights and accommodation and got involved with as much as possible. I went out for beers with people, met loads of people and I remember saying to myself "I've got nothing to lose". I don't think everyone is prepared to go out and network and meet people. I'm not saying you must go to conferences, but you must be brave enough to reach out to people. That certainly helped me along my way and it's important if you're trying to get into sport nutrition.

Who would have thought that our friendship together started over a beer at ISENC! What's been the biggest challenge of your career today?

Marcus: The workload can be difficult and challenging. Having a big workload means you have to work long hours; you've got to work weekends and make sacrifices. I have a lot of friends that work 9–5 jobs and they can go out every weekend. They always ask me to come out for beers or join them for activities this weekend. You can't always do it, so I think some of the sacrifices and hard work have probably been some of the biggest challenges.

During the three years that I was at Everton Football Club we collected longitudinal data, body composition and resting metabolic rate (RMR). As you are aware, RMR data must be collected in the morning when fasted (i.e. no food or fluid ingested). Therefore, this was collected during the school holidays because we could not take the kids out of school in the morning to collect the data. Over this three-year period, during all the school holidays, I was in university with the players collecting the data. I only ever took two days off for Christmas at a time, which was tough, because I had to be in scanning and assessing the players and getting it done for my PhD. However, they are sacrifices you must make, just as you have done, and as many others have done. You've got to be prepared to do that.

What characteristics do you think people need to work in the industry of performance nutrition?

Marcus: Good question. A lot of the people working in some of the top jobs in sport nutrition around the UK have PhDs, and more practitioners are getting PhDs. I personally think that's the way it's moving forward as it allows you to set yourself apart from others. I don't know how many sport science, nutrition or dietetics students are graduating each year, but having only a BSc degree qualification isn't enough anymore. Students have to now have a master's as a bare minimum, but I give it another 5–10 years and you will need a PhD if you are to have a chance at being successful in your application for the top jobs. Obviously, you've got to work hard, you've got to be prepared to make sacrifices to get to that stage and I think you also must have the right character and be the right person.

If you want to be in sports nutrition or be a performance nutritionist, whether that's working with individual athletes, or in a team environment, you must be a people person. Now I have a squad of about 30 players, all different ages, experiences, nationalities, so you must be able to get on with them, communicate and work in an environment which is very fluid, dynamic and with lots of different characters, egos and personalities. So, I think having people skills is certainly another big skill that people should ensure they have.

What would be your biggest recommendation to your younger self or to aspiring students entering the industry now?

Marcus: Go and get experience. I don't need to say it; it's obvious you need your education and qualifications. You need an MSc at minimum if you want to become a Sport and Exercise Nutrition Register (SENr) accredited nutritionist. It goes without saying, you need experience and people need to be smart. Some MSc courses offer experience during the course, but you need to go above and beyond that. You need to get experience earlier during your undergraduate years. If you're going to take time away from studies, that's fine, but again you need to get experience and it doesn't have to be at Premier League level.

People want to see that you're interacting with people, you are offering advice, you are getting in and amongst it. For me, it also tells me a little bit about your personality: "This person is being proactive and going out and trying to get some experience". Yes, it might be a job with a Sunday League team (lower football division) but at least you're being proactive and showing a willingness, to do what many can't be bothered to do! I've had placement students in the past who work with me. They do the placement and sort of think "Oh well that's brilliant, I'll go get a job now" and that's the end of it. I've offered other bits of work, advice and placement opportunities and they don't want to do it. But unfortunately, you've got to do it.

Are there areas that you didn't learn on the course that have been important for you now that you're working full time?

Marcus: The behaviour change area, particularly in the context of sport nutrition. I do think that will become integrated into MSc courses. Coaching and the ability to coach well is certainly an important aspect too. I'm a foodie; I love food and will play about with food recipes but one of the things that I have seen in sports nutrition, or more in the sport science route, is that some people don't have a good understanding of food and nutrients. This is an area which can be practically developed. It's all well and good developing meal plans, yes, the classic chicken and pasta which everyone prescribes in nutrition strategies, but how can you be a bit more creative, using a wider variety of foods?

Where do you think the future of nutrition will be in five years' time? Considering you have just started working full time with professional football players, are there any little areas you're beginning to see that might progress nutrition forward?

Marcus: It will be individualised with more full-time practitioners. I think we've probably seen over the last five years, a transition from the consultancy model, maybe a day a month to a day a week, to two days per week. You're now seeing more full-time positions and I think give it another five years, I think the consultancy model will be no more, as people realise the importance and impact of nutritionists in the building. Organisations will get more out of it if they recruit full-time practitioners in the club who can build better relationship with individual players.

Cannabidiol is a hot topic; I know there's more research going on in this area. One of the other things as well, I'm still not convinced practitioners are consistently implementing things well. I think that translation from research into practice is huge. I think we as practitioners can get better at how we translate the information to the athletes.

Is there a book that you've read recently which has improved your practice? This doesn't have to be nutrition related, this could just be anything that you've read recently or doesn't have to be a book, but even an article?

Marcus: I've been reading mainly autobiographies, so to be honest, nothing that's changed my practice. One book I have read twice is *Deep Work* by Cal Newport. I wouldn't say it changes day-to-day nutrition practice, but it's changed the way I work during my days off or when working on research projects. Working in the evenings or on my days off, it was a good book to re-read. Some key things he talks about are efficiency and distraction from work. There's some good stuff in that book. Reading of the scientific literature is so important for us as practitioners. You practise your knowledge from this, and you tweak things within your practice each day from the updated literature.

Are there any key principles that you try to follow every day or are there things that you have started bringing into your daily lifestyle that you may not have done when we first met?

Marcus: Routine is important. I like it and I think I'm at my best when I'm in a good routine. I go to bed early, I get up early, but they're generally pretty set times: 10pm and 6am. I make sure I get good sleep and try to exercise most days, as this helps look after my general well-being. If you look after yourself everything else should fall into place. I think reflections are important too. I know people reflect in different ways. Some people like to write it down, although personally I struggle to do this. Instead, I will ring people, have a good call and chew the fat, get their opinion on things. That's how I reflect. Occasionally, I will note things down. It doesn't have to be every day, or even every week, but I think when something of note happens, I will write it down. I think if you can build reflections into your routine, it will be massive. It's something I should do more myself.

Finally, probably the golden question, what makes a successful performance nutritionist?

Marcus: Certainly, someone that knows the science for the context they are working in. So, for example, you and I have both worked in football and so I think to be successful, the first step is knowing the football literature, physiology and nutrition and the wider football literature inside out. This is important; you could have a conversation at any time or any location with anyone. You need to know that information at the top of your head. I've got players that aren't very well educated so we start with basics, but I have some players where I have quite high-level conversations. These conversations will just happen, it could be in the canteen, it could be crossing each other in the corridor.

I think having the people skills, emotional intelligence and communications skills is key, alongside a good work ethic. When you work in professional sport as you'll be aware, it's not really a 9–5 job. You must be prepared to pick up the phone at 10 o'clock at night, or for someone ringing you on your days off. Working in professional sport is more of a lifestyle.

MY REFLECTIONS FROM MARCUS'S INTERVIEW

The first thing that I took away from this interview is how bold Marcus has been to reach out to people at all stages of his career. If he hadn't contacted Oxford United Football Club, he would not have gained any experience at this stage of his career. I also admire him for attending ISENC on his own, flying over to the conference, not knowing anyone, which can be a little intimidating. However, I am personally very happy he did as this is where we met and started our friendship together.

Having witnessed Marcus first-hand navigate his way through his PhD and the relentless hours of hard work he put into it, it is no surprise that he repeatedly mentions the importance of working hard to be successful. Studying an applied PhD can be tricky at times, however staying focused on the task at hand and the journey can be an enjoyable one. I have also read the book *Deep Work* and would highly recommend it for those people who find themselves a little distracted at times.

Finally, I resonate well with Marcus's final point about reading and knowing the literature in your area. I was also taught by Professors James Morton and Graeme Close to always be able to answer three whys to any question asked of you by an athlete. For example, why is protein important, why should we consume it and why does it help muscles?

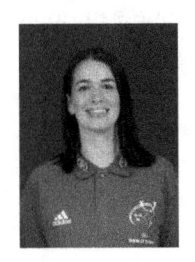

CHAPTER 6:
DR EMMA TESTER

Emma currently works as the Lead Performance Nutritionist (maternity cover) for Tottenham Hotspur Football Club. Emma has previous experience as an academy nutritionist at Leicester City Football Club and more recently almost five years as the Lead Performance Nutritionist at Munster Rugby Club in Ireland. Emma studied her undergraduate degree in Sport and Exercise Science at Leeds Metropolitan University, her Master's degree in Sport and Exercise Nutrition at Leeds Beckett University and PhD in Optimising Recovery in Rugby League Players at Leeds Beckett University.

Emma and I have only ever met once in person, at the International Sport and Exercise Nutrition Conference. Since then, we have always kept a close eye on what each other is doing in the industry and have often exchanged messages via social media platforms to help each other out.

You can follow Emma on Twitter @testeremma

Emma, for those who don't know you, could you just give a quick background as to who you are and your experience?

Emma: I studied my sport science undergraduate degree in 2006. I picked this study area because I was good at PE, which is why a lot of people decide to take this path. However, a lot of universities have many course options available now and it's important for people to pick a more specific route.

It probably wasn't until my third year that I realised that it was sport nutrition I wanted to study. The modules and topics for sport nutrition were great, and I was good at it, so I carried this on into my master's. All of my study years were at Leeds Beckett University. Their sports nutrition course was one of the first in the UK that achieved the Sport and Exercise Nutrition Register (SENr) status. Louise Sutton was the programme lead and she had a huge involvement in setting up SENr.

It was a good course and other institutions caught up with similar course content. For example, when I did the internship programme, there were two of us in the same position for the year. It was basically a one-on-one personal training system to support nutrition practitioners developing their practical nutrition skills. It was such great exposure, and I was lucky to get it. At the time, I didn't have any nutrition or sport science experience – apart from two weeks' work experience when I shadowed my school PE teacher – and because I did not have any experience, I worked my arse off to get the internship.

Every opportunity that was presented to me in university, I agreed to do it. I was trying to work with all the nutritional related projects that were going on at the time, with lots of the local teams. Leeds as a city is a great place for the sport side of things. All the local teams were involved with the university. Cricket, both rugby codes, swimmers; we even had the Team Great Britain racewalking and lifting teams based at Leeds. With Team GB lifting, I managed to do an internship with them which was amazing. I was working with future Olympic racewalkers and potential Olympic lifters. The spread of sports and exposure I got was outstanding. It was a bit of everything. It gave me a good and very broad understanding of what athletes are like, how you work with them, and how to engage with lots of different types of people. All the athletes were very different in various ways.

I stayed on at the university, and worked as a nutrition project officer, mentoring the next year of internship students who progressed through the university. This involved working on the same sports and groups, but now in a paid role. It was great and it was a good way to learn. It involved teaching and helping others to develop, which in turn allowed me to keep developing. I still do a bit of self-development now. I observe others and then apply it to my own practice whilst providing opportunities for other people to observe me as well. This has been beneficial for me because I've been in my current role now for quite a few years. Personally, my own continuing professional development is visiting other clubs, going in and seeing or speaking to other practitioners who are doing similar and to see what I can learn.

During my current role, I also started my PhD. I was self-funding it originally and it started off with a focus on recovery in rugby players. Like many applied PhDs, it has taken me a long time, but then again, I must remind myself I moved to another country and set up another life at the same time. I moved to Munster in 2016 and I have been with the full-time senior squad for 4–5 years.

When you say you moved there, you mean you moved to Ireland to work with Munster?

Emma: That's right. I remember when I told people that I had got a job and was moving to Ireland. A lot of people in the UK don't realise that Ireland is another country, that they have a different currency, and they speak Irish. A lot of people underestimated how big a deal it was to move, even though it is close to England and just over a very choppy sea.

When would you say was the first time you were directly involved in nutrition?

Emma: As an actual practitioner it was during my MSc year. A lot of people on my course had more experience than me. However, I am the only one from my year group who is a practitioner working in sport now. I took every opportunity. I felt I was a "yes" person in my first few years. Every opportunity that was presented to me, it was a yes!

Much of that experience early on would have been volunteering, wouldn't it?

Emma: Yes, most of it. I had three internships happening in the year after my MSc, and I also started the paid role within the university. Then I went to Leicester City Football Club for a season as an internship student. I did a good job and they kept me on for two more seasons in a paid consultancy role. There is quite a lot of controversy about paid versus unpaid work. At the time, it wasn't possible to get into the system and gain experience without doing something for nothing. However, it wasn't for nothing. It was all the experience you gained, all the mentorship you received, which almost offset not getting paid.

At Leeds Beckett University, if you were selected as an internship, you actually got half your course fees paid which was amazing. This was a long time ago when course fees aren't the price they are now, but it massively helped. Nowadays we should try and source more paid work at an internship level, even if it is to cover things like expenses. Clubs have money. For example, in my role now, I managed to set up a small internship post that had some money attached to it. I managed to set it up in a way that utilised some money that we had from our supplement sponsor and some internal money to help part fund it. It wasn't large amounts of money from one place, it was a contribution from many places, and moving forward we have to be smart about how we put together this type of role.

I remember when I started my MSc there was this bad stigma around supplements and nutrition companies etc. They were seen as something to stay away from, almost. Hopefully now with all the awareness around supplement safety, that should be gone. Even utilising meal prep companies to help support and fund some of these positions is a great idea. It can be done; I've done it, and many others have done it – I'm not the first! If we offer the funding company something in return, for example writing articles, analysing meals or recipes then both parties are happy.

We need to be better at finding financial support for future practitioners, otherwise we are going to be in the same boat where people will be doing something for nothing for a long time before they are able to have enough experience behind them to get a paid job. When you look at other career paths it's insane, individuals with MScs or PhDs doing work for nothing; it just wouldn't happen. We can drive that change and it's important we do so.

Who are some of the biggest mentors in your life and why have they been so important to you?

Emma: In the academic and sport world, Louise Sutton from the MSc programme at Leeds Beckett. She was my first mentor, helping me learn how to reflect, how to develop and teach others. When I came to Munster, I then started working with Aled Walters and he really had my back. He was the first person (outside of nutrition) who had my corner. He let me explore and let me be the expert; instead of telling me how it should be done, he let me have control of the nutrition provision. Then Ruth Wood-Martin from the Irish Rugby Football Union. Ruth is a phenomenal practitioner. She has managed to set up an entire nutrition system within Irish rugby and now all the provinces have access to at least one nutritionist, but most have access to two. Considering there are four provinces, she has done a great job setting up the entire system.

As for everyone, the period of COVID-19 has been incredibly challenging, but Ruth is a really supportive person, and she finds things challenging too. It's nice to know that we are not on our own and others are going through challenges and problems too. Outside of the work environment, my friends are supportive. Having that ability to switch off, I think my friendship group are probably the best people to do that with. I don't know whether it's mentorship with your friends, but it teaches you how to switch off and be a normal person.

What's been a standout moment for you in your career to date?

Emma: It isn't an achievement but more of a moment. We were in the semi-final of the European Rugby Cup and there were 50,000 Munster fans singing "The Fields of Athenry" all at the same time. I was thinking to myself, don't get distracted; I can't take it when they start singing; it's so emotional and I need to concentrate on my job. I remember being on the side of the pitch and looking around at one of the players and we were both close to tears, it must have been about 50th minute in the match. It was just incredible. It wasn't an achievement moment, but I just thought, wow, people really give a s**t about this club, like they really love being here. That's probably one of my standout moments where you realise you are just a small part of something so big.

It makes you realise how powerful sport can be, doesn't it, people paying for the tickets and spending money, all for the love of rugby?

Emma: Yeah, I agree, and I think even now (due to COVID-19) people can't do normal things. I feel really privileged that I can carry on doing my work. For some people it is an outlet for them. To have something to look forward to, something they love and some form of entertainment, it is important. It really matters to people.

Going from your days of being an internship student at Leeds Beckett University, to now leading sports nutrition at Munster, this is a successful career. What do you think have been the most influential factors as to why you have had your success in your career so far?

Emma: It's because I am really determined. As I have got older, I have become more confident in my ability to challenge things that I do not think are right in and around the work setting. If I think there is a different approach or way of doing something, I will speak up. I have heard stories of where backroom staff like nutritionists don't get treated with the respect they deserve.

When you are younger, you are so keen to be there, you will be the person that says yes to everything, and you do anything. Whereas now, I always assess and think, is the way you are speaking to me acceptable or is what you are asking me to do acceptable or not, and if not, how do we come to a solution for it?

One of the things I know I am good at, is trying to find solutions. If I don't like something, I am not going to moan, I will look for the other option that might be available. I will do this until I reach a point of compromise. I don't easily give in.

We have an academy role now, and if I see someone treating this position in a way that is unacceptable then I will raise this. It's hard; there is such a spectrum to how clubs operate. Some operate in silo, some work as a collective. I have found at some clubs, people want to take a complete lead on nutrition, but it may not be what they are there to do. In nutrition we are taught about professional practice and it's a big part of the SENr accreditation process, learning and understanding where the limits of your practice are. However, I don't think this process is embedded well in other disciplines. For example, if the club does not have a nutritionist, then the strength and conditioning coach will often take control over nutrition practice at the club. However, this would be frowned upon if it was the other way around! Therefore, challenging this is something I try to do.

I do try and reflect on where I have been and where I am. Sometimes when you are in it, you forget where you have come from. Even when you are having a bad time, reflect and take a second to think you are proud of what you have done and where you have got to and where you will go to. These are little things about myself that I think have helped me get to the point I am at now.

Aligned to those tougher times, what do you think has been the biggest challenge of your career to date?

Emma: In my current career as a nutritionist, people often ask me the question: "What is it like to work in a male-dominated environment?" I always respond to say, it is male majority, but it is not male dominated. I'm not dominated in work at all. There are people who like to dictate and that is where it can be challenging at times, but that's also where perseverance pays off.

I am lucky, at the Ireland Rugby Football Union, there's a whole system of nutritionists. There are about 10 of us, so to have 10 brains to call on, to share experiences and to ask advice on certain things, is great. It is something that does help, and it would have been a lot harder for me if I didn't have anyone working with me, but we all work as a team. Even through COVID-19 we have continued to have Zoom calls every week. We have continued to do this every other week, even now that we have all been back in our facilities since June or July 2020.

Professional sport can be challenging at times, especially if there is a high staff turnover. If you get someone who is quite a dominating character, then that can be challenging. I've seen a few staff leave the last few years and they may have been great. Then you get someone new, and you have to go through that whole process again, building the relationship, understanding each other's boundaries, how you are going to work together. I think this is where sport can be unique in a way, a high turnover of staff in a short number of years. Ultimately, you are dealing with people and that's always challenging. Everything else, if you are a solution-focused person, then everything is possible.

What characteristics do you think people need to work in performance nutrition?

Emma: Coming from one angle of working in male team sports, you do have to be resilient. I've known other great practitioners who have given up because it wasn't for them or it's been too much for them, which is a shame when it's something they were passionate about. You need to be resilient, but you also need to challenge what isn't right. Everyone is different, and everyone should have their own personality. You don't have to be the bubbly person in the room. You must have a bit of give and take and you've got to be able to have a laugh with them.

If you're just starting out in your career and you're not the most confident person in the room, you don't have to be. It's not often that you're going to be a practitioner in front of loads of people all at once. Some of the more meaningful conversations will be the one-to-ones. If you can relate to people, you're going to get more out of that than being the one who is stood in the middle of the pitch or in the gym shouting. I don't necessarily think *the* personality matters; if you've got *a* personality, it doesn't really matter what kind of one it is.

Attention to detail, that's something that some people don't have. When you're delivering a specific message and you haven't noticed a mistake, or a group session that you're running, to me, it really makes the difference between something good or something that is average. You might be a good practitioner nailing your work, but if you've got poor attention to detail, it's going to contribute to errors. It happened to me when I was previously supervising some master's students; they would miss an entire meal or an entire line out of someone's food diary analysis. They basically missed out 500 calories' worth of analysis! Everything you do and your conclusions off the back of this analysis is going to be wrong. Personally, people must have attention to detail; it's important.

A lot of people have a fear of failure. I've seen it with people; it stops you doing anything at all because of how you may be perceived by others around you. So, they don't do anything or it limits how much they do. I think this is important for more inexperienced people.

These are the qualities that I look for, more so than how much experience they have got or how much education they've got. If they have ticked the criteria-based stuff, it's then the finer detail. When you receive loads of CVs, I check to see if they have followed the instructions and sent in a one-page CV. We had an internship post-out a couple years ago now and someone had a longer CV than me. They had just written everything they could in there. It was far too long; I asked for a one-page CV, and you sent me seven. It's attention to details with things like this; I think it is important, but people forget about it.

What would be your biggest recommendation to your younger self or to aspiring students entering the industry now?

Emma: Take opportunities that arise but also know your worth. You might have to do a bit of work for free, but you shouldn't spend your whole career doing things without being paid. I get it even now; people ask could you just answer a quick couple of questions on XYZ, how do I make something like this taste good, how do you establish someone's protein intake, how do I ensure I get the body I want?

There are many job specifications available that you could look at and see what you may need to get that job in the future. Create a plan for when you're going to achieve the things you are missing. It's easy to think you must do everything in one go. For example, you may be thinking you must have your food hygiene certificate, your qualification to allow you to do skinfold measurements, your United Kingdom Anti-Doping qualification. Although you do have to have it all, you do not need to overwhelm yourself and try and do it all at once. For example, I only recently completed my high-performance Sport and Exercise Nutrition Practitioner registration and it's 2020. I have always had other things to do at the same time, but it's always been there and something that I have always needed to do. Plan it out; don't feel like you must do everything all in the next year and especially in the year straight after graduating. It's just not going to be possible and don't berate yourself for not having got it done immediately.

Being yourself is something that is important. Someone provided some feedback from a workshop that I had done once and said to my supervisor, "She just needs to smile more!" I thought that's not helpful, but I've still managed to get a fair way along a career path without apparently being a smiling person. I suggest being yourself and ignore people trolling you. Read a lot and read quite broadly. That will help you develop an interest in an area and then you can become more proficient in that area. Reading broadly also keeps you aware of what's going on outside of your little bubble too.

Reading is a big area to consider when you're working as a full-time practitioner. It's very easy to get frustrated that you may not have read anything for a couple of weeks, and it's important to set yourself time in the week for dedicated reading.

Emma: I've only got through my reading pile once in the last 10 years. It was because of extra time that the COVID lockdowns provided me, but otherwise I've always got something that's in my little reading pile.

Are there areas that you did not learn on the course that have been important for you considering you are now working full time?

Emma: As I said before, the Leeds Beckett University course was one of the first to become accredited, so having an applied practice programme back then was very rare. Without this I wouldn't have known the breadth of topics that I know. There are of course many I am still learning! However, more courses now have elements of the practitioner programme, which back when I was studying would have been the most difficult thing to have got hold of. I was lucky that I got the internship position and that's potentially why I am the only one from that year group who is a practitioner. Not everyone had the exposure or experience back then. Whereas as the course developed at Leeds Becket University, they changed it from having just a one-person internship, to a couple of people, to a small cohort, then to everyone on the course having the opportunity to engage in professional practice.

Again, I would re-emphasise how important it is to read things beyond the course itself. Having taught and delivered lectures for quite a long time, I can say this with confidence. A lot of students read what they need to read so they can pass the exam and then it stops, instead of reading quite broadly and then developing an interest in something specific. I feel like the students that read more are able to engage more in sessions and discuss things to a greater detail and suggest different ideas, whereas the ones who just read to pass the exam couldn't go far with their discussions.

Where do you think the future of nutrition will be in five years' time?

Emma: Hopefully more full-time roles and opportunities, but like I said at the start, I think that's down to people like you and I to help create these roles. So maybe in five years' time, anyone in an employed position would be offering further work to someone else, whether it's a full-time position or even just a small placement. We should also be pushing younger practitioners to have older practitioners as mentors. You really do learn a lot from that process, and it reminds you of the stuff that you learned years ago but now haven't looked at for a while. Essentially more jobs and more intelligence on how we fund these positions.

The mentoring side of things is a big area and I've enjoyed running my mentorship programme recently. Is there a book that you've recently read which has improved your practice?

Emma: I've read more recipe books which sounds weird but there are only so many vegetables a rugby player will eat. I have got a series of three of the Bosh vegetarian and vegan cookbooks because they know how to do vegetables well. Instead of just steamed broccoli there is a lot more we can do. A big part of my practice is the menu design, what recipes can we do. We don't have a performance chef, so it's all coming from myself. Being able to give the caterers ideas is crucial.

Have you read a book outside of nutrition recently?

Emma: The Barack Obama autobiography. It's interesting on how he interacts with colleagues, staff and people that he is having to work with. Some of the stuff he says is the same type of scenario that goes on in sport; it's all leadership content that we all read about and it's interesting that even the ex-president of America and lead sports nutritionists are facing the same challenges, but on a slightly different scale!

Are there any key principles that you try to follow every day?

Emma: I don't know if it's a daily thing but especially when I was writing up my PhD and when I moved here, I was like "Just get it done, just get s**t done!" Sometimes you don't want to do something, but I just had to get it done and then move on to the next thing. That's my daily approach.

My dad used to say to me that Nike's logo sums it up: "Just Do It". Obviously, you have to think about stuff, and you have to plan and prepare, but at the end of the day just do it, just get it done.

Finally, in your eyes, what makes a successful performance nutritionist?

Emma: Someone who knows their stuff and knows how to apply it, but also knows how to get people on board with the application. Everyone's aware of the theory and how important the practical application is, but it's also how well you get the person to do what you want them to do. It's the behaviour change area that becomes important. You can apply content and you can make things available, but unless someone buys into what you're trying to sell it's not effective practice. Someone who knows their stuff, knows how to apply it, and can get people on board.

MY REFLECTIONS FROM EMMA'S INTERVIEW

Although Emma openly admits that she had to do free volunteering experience in her early years, I love the way she reframes this as clear applied practice. There are many students who struggle to grasp the concept that a little bit of experience could be highly valuable for them later in their career.

Emma has been clever with the way she has recycled some of the money from supplement sponsors into paid placement projects within the club and I agree with her, I think this is what the experienced practitioners should all be aiming to achieve now. It is a great way to provide junior practitioners with the opportunity to gain experience but also ensure they are paid for their time.

Finally, an area that I think is very important for younger practitioners who are entering the industry now to understand and realise, is to have a social circle and interests outside of their chosen sport or career path. The ability to switch off from work and come back again another day with fresh eyes and a rested mind can result in highly efficient and effective work.

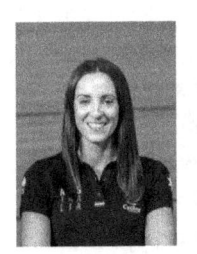

CHAPTER 7:
DR JILL LECKEY

Since November 2017, Jill has worked with Cycling Australia as a performance nutritionist. Prior to this role, Jill spent one year with the Malaysian Track Cycling team in 2015–2016 before spending a year with Melbourne Football Club in 2017.

I first met Jill when I was studying my undergraduate degree at LJMU. Jill was a few years ahead of me in the university, having studied her undergraduate degree in Sport Science from 2008–2011 and then her MSc degree in Sports Physiology from 2011–2012. Jill then moved to Australia to study her PhD at the Australian Catholic University from 2014–2017 titled "Exercise-nutrient interactions: Effects on substrate metabolism and performance".

You can follow Jill on Twitter @Jill_Leckey

Jill, could you give an insight into who you are and what your background is?

Jill: I was born and bred in Belfast, Ireland and spent the first 18 years of my life there before moving to Liverpool to go to university. I was always a sporty, active child and my favourite sport was athletics. I remember looking at university courses with my family and them saying "What do you love doing, what do you enjoy?" I knew that I loved sport, biology, physical education and maths. I looked at sport science and criminology courses; these seemed fitting because I always thought I wanted to be in the police! I ended up choosing sport science and I moved to Liverpool to study a Bachelor of Sport Science at LJMU in 2008. At the time, I did not think about where I would be after my studies; it was more about doing something I really loved. Right now, I am currently living in Australia, working for the Australian Cycling Team.

How and when did you first get involved in nutrition?

Jill: During the sport science course at LJMU, I always chose the nutrition and physiology subjects as I enjoyed these the most. Unfortunately, I did not enjoy the psychology and biomechanics subjects and dropped these when I could! My love for the other subjects was influenced by several lecturers at LJMU, who were passionate about what they were teaching, and it really connected with me. I saw the link early on in my studies with how nutrition could support athletes day to day with training and adaptation. During the course, there were also a few case studies shared about the lecturers' personal journeys and how they managed to get into sport clubs. This really made me excited. I remember the exercise metabolism unit; it was interesting and fascinating. Following my undergraduate degree, I completed the Master's in Sports Physiology at LJMU, and several of the units were focused on nutrition. In support of the studies, I also did a couple of placements with football clubs and a swimming club. I remember going into the clubs and chatting to the athletes and their parents about nutrition support for training sessions. It is quite funny looking back on it all now, to be honest.

You've progressed from the football and swimming club years ago to where you are now. Walk me through your nutrition career after that. Speaking to you right now, I can see a great backdrop and you're obviously sitting there in a nice sunny environment.

Jill: After my master's, I moved back to Belfast for a short period and during that time I bought a road bike. The idea of buying a road bike was from my parents; I think they wanted to ensure I stayed sane while living at home again. I did a few group rides and as you can imagine, I got my nutrition as wrong as you could possibly get it, which was a good learning curve. After six months at home, I started a role with an endurance sports nutrition company, who I worked with for a year.

It was an interesting process. When I got interviewed for the role, they didn't think I had enough experience for the job, which was understandable just coming out of my master's. I then got rejected for the job. I was disappointed as I saw this as the perfect job for me. I went back to them and proposed that they give me a short-term trial and if they didn't feel I was suited to the job, then they could let me go. I explained to the company that when you have just finished university, it's difficult if companies are only looking for individuals with experience. They were really open to my proposal, which was great, and they gave me the opportunity.

During this role, I engaged with other practitioners and researchers in the nutrition industry, and I was beginning to realise that if I really wanted to succeed, I needed a PhD. After speaking to the lecturers at LJMU and asking what a PhD consisted of, I decided I really wanted to do one (upon reflection, I am not sure I truly understood what it was).

It was recommended that I email the researchers whose papers I enjoyed reading. I remember thinking to myself, who would ever reply to me; no one knows who I am! I knew I had nothing to lose, so I emailed Professor Louise Burke at the Australian Institute of Sport and she suggested I email Professor John Hawley, as my skillset would align with his research better. John also responded to my email and once we clarified that I matched the requirements (a first-class honours degree and a minimum of one publication), we went back and forth for many months while waiting to see if any scholarship opportunities became available within his university. I should mention that John was based in Melbourne, Australia.

Eventually an opportunity became available and quite quickly I was interviewed and offered a four-year scholarship. During the wait, I had an interview for a different PhD, which would have taken my career on a completely different path. The other PhD was in protein metabolism with the elderly population, so life could have been very different to what it is now!

Although I was excited for the new chapter, I was gutted to leave the UK and the job I was in. I moved to Melbourne, and I spent three and a half years there. When I moved over to Melbourne, I didn't know anyone (thankfully my sister lived in Sydney), so I was almost starting from scratch again, and had to build up a good network. During that time, the research I was conducting focused on endurance exercise and metabolism. This was exactly the topic I wanted to study, and I was really fascinated in how nutrition could have such an impact on prolonged exercise.

During my PhD, I taught laboratory tutorials at the university, and did some lectures. I also made it known to a few people that I was really interested in sport and asked them how I could get into the industry. I met Dr Stuart Cormack who was a lecturer and a high-performance consultant for several sports at the time. I made it known to him that I was interested in sport and keen to get involved in any opportunities that came up. Whether that meant shadowing a dietitian, or standing on the sidelines shaking protein shakes, whatever it was, I was willing to do it.

Stu opened the door to a few opportunities. One was with an Olympic track cyclist in Melbourne, so this was a very exciting opportunity, to observe and work alongside the dietitian. Also, Stu managed to help me secure work at an Australian rules football club. I also was fortunate enough to have Professor Louise Burke as one of my PhD supervisors and was able to spend some time helping on a research study at the Australian Institute of Sport and completed one of my own research studies there, with an elite cycling team. These opportunities and experiences sealed the deal on realising that I was committed to finding a career within elite sport.

Towards the end of the PhD, I was convinced I was going to end up working in football because that's where the opportunity was at the time. However, I found out the Australian Cycling Team were recruiting for a nutritionist and the timing was perfect. I finished the PhD and within three months I had started the new role as the Performance Nutritionist with the Australian national track cycling team. When I applied for the role, I didn't know where they were based, which is ridiculous, but it all happened quite quickly. It turned out that they were based in Adelaide, which is about an hour's flight from Melbourne or a 10-hour drive. I packed my bags and moved to Adelaide.

So, when you landed in Adelaide, you literally had to start your network again. Was it like "I'm on my own again and let's see what happens"?

Jill: I remember packing up my car, starting the drive and thinking to myself, "What are you doing, I am absolutely nuts". I had a car full of stuff and I didn't know anyone that lived in Adelaide. It really did feel like I was starting again. However, I had people in my life who had been very supportive through all the ups and downs of the PhD and one of these people was Professor James Morton. I am incredibly grateful for all his support throughout my studies and career to date.

It was a fresh start in a new role; at the time I only knew two dietitians in Australia (of which one was Professor Louise Burke). I did think how on earth was I going to build a network of people for myself. It has taken time, but I have put a lot of work into reaching out to people, asking questions and sharing information. Australia has sports institutes in each state and if you were to drive around them all, it would take you about 80 hours, and that's probably only a third of the country. It's a big country so you don't always get to meet people in person. Thankfully, the cycling team were very supportive during my move and gave me time to settle into the role and find my feet. I am very grateful for this.

You touched on it a little bit, but who are your mentors and why have they been important in your life?

Jill: First and foremost, my family and parents who have been a massive support network the whole way through studying and working. They fully supported my move to Australia for the PhD and were keen for me to spread my wings and continue learning. Having them on the other side of the phone and always pushing me forward has been amazing. They are not afraid of hard work and instilled this in me from a young age. We joke about just getting on with it (or at least they tell me that), and I think that's just part of being from Belfast; you just get stuck in and work hard.

In addition to my parents, as I said Professor James Morton has been a huge influence and support. I first met James during my undergraduate degree and 11 years later, I still hassle him for advice. When I moved to Melbourne, I asked him if he would be happy to be involved in my PhD as an additional supervisor and he was willing to do that. I really respect James as he tells me the truth; he is honest and has the hard conversations that are sometimes needed. He brings me back in line when needed and has also often pulled me out of challenging times.

As I mentioned, Dr Stuart McCormack and Professors Louise Burke and John Hawley have also been integral in my career to date. I remember when I told Stuart that I got offered the job with cycling, he looked at a poster on his wall which was from the Sydney 2000 Olympic Games and he said, "That was one of the best moments of my life and I hope you get to experience it one day". I've never forgotten that moment.

Has there been a standout moment in your career to date?

Jill: I attended the World Championships in 2019 with the cycling team. The team came home with quite a few rainbow jerseys (winning jersey); it was a very successful event. Being part of a winning team and realising that you're an important cog in the team is an exciting realisation. There have been some key moments of simply sitting in meetings with the whole multidisciplinary team and thinking to myself, we are planning for the Olympics Games; this is as big as it gets in elite sport. Then thinking,

I cannot believe that I'm sitting here with coaches, physiotherapists, doctors and discussing athletes who have been to many Olympic Games, Commonwealth Games and World Championship events. I remember when I was a young student, hearing in lectures that if I worked in sport, it would be with a multidisciplinary team and in those moments thinking, this is it! This is what everyone talked about. For sure, I think some of those Olympic planning meetings make you realise why we do what we do!

I've interviewed Dr Marcus Hannon and Dr Dan Martin and they both said similar. Sometimes it's not the winning of the match or the medal, but it's more being in those moments of listening to a manager give the team talk. Sometimes I have thought to myself, am I sitting in here with a squad of players that are worth £X million and I'm listening to the team talk by the manager? Even moments that I have been fortunate to experience, like walking out at Wembley with your team for the Challenge Cup Final with your mum, dad and brothers in the crowd. Being able to go and see them at the end of the game in the crowd, these are special moments.

Moving on, what do you think has been the most influential factor as to why you've had your successes so far in your career?

Jill: I am very driven and motivated to succeed. I don't need external motivation to get me out of bed in the morning. I'm also keen on setting myself goals and constantly looking at how I can improve. Even in the job that I currently have, I'm constantly thinking how we can break through barriers and find ways to improve things. I have always been open to opportunities. I've been prepared to move across the world, move states, take risks, jump right in and see what happens. I've also worked hard to surround myself with good people and build a strong network wherever I have been. So, I think being determined, open to opportunities and having self-belief, but also having people to support me when I do have those doubts.

Having important people behind you when moments get a little tough is very important! What would you say has been the biggest challenge in your career to date?

Jill: I don't think I have one specific moment, however one of the biggest challenges is influencing stakeholders. When you think of high-performance programmes, nutrition is one element in the whole programme, and it can't always be the priority. I know sometimes I can almost feel a bit defeated or deflated when my ideas regarding nutrition do not get over the line and are not implemented straight away. Additionally, learning how to work with a diverse range of stakeholders within an organisation can be challenging.

A big thing that happened for us all in the last couple of years was the *Game Changers* programme which was aired on Netflix. When that was shown on TV, many people at the time were slamming meat and dairy. On one hand it was amazing as it ignited some brilliant conversations around the dinner table but it also uncovered people's lack of education around fundamental nutrition. Did it come up in any conversations within your work?

Jill: Yes, it was at the forefront of people's minds, but sometimes these things are an enjoyable challenge. In this situation it was easy to predict what questions might be asked and you can plan how best to respond to them. I would also add the fact that we are all in the same industry, and I can pick up the phone to you and ask you if you are having the same issues. There are always people to talk to about it.

What characteristics do you think people need to work in the industry of performance nutrition?

Jill: You do have to be driven, motivated and determined to succeed. Sport is not an easy industry to get into, so being driven to network and communicate with people is key. You need to be resilient because in sport, the highs are high, and the successes are great when you're in a winning team, but when it doesn't go to plan, the morale can be low. Ultimately, in my role, I try and be the stable person in the team whether the morale is high or not. The way you deal with problems says a lot about who you are as well. Always be prepared to improve yourself; I don't mean change who you are, but you must be prepared to understand yourself better and receive feedback on what others perceive of you. This can be confronting at times but is highly rewarding.

If you go back to yourself 10 years ago, what would be your biggest recommendation to your younger self or to students entering the industry now?

Jill: Say yes to opportunities that arise and back yourself to do them well. Sharing your aspirations with someone is key because all you need is one person to take a chance on you and give you an opportunity which could change your life. In my eyes, you create your own luck, so go out there and talk to people about your ideas. Another key point is to look after your own health and well-being. I have found this to be key in the whole process; if you don't look after yourself, no one else will. Other people will care, but ultimately it comes down to you to really look after the mind and body.

Some students are not willing to say yes to the opportunities if they're not paid. The amount of volunteering that I did was an investment in myself. I did a full year at Saracens Rugby Club, St Helens Rugby Club. Every Saturday morning at 07:00, I would take my bike and get on the train from Liverpool to St Helens to help at the club. I did this for free, but I did it because I knew the experience was key. It's part of the problem that I see with students who are graduating with degrees. Some graduate and expect to be employed straight away.

That isn't how the cookie crumbles, unfortunately. Saying yes to opportunities and taking those opportunities is important.

Jill: There are only a certain number of national teams, and each team is well established in a specific location, so you do have to move for the role sometimes. Of course, there are certain times in life where you may not be able to move, but I think when you can, you must jump at the opportunity. It can be risky, and it can be scary. I think back to driving to Adelaide and saying to myself "What are you doing?", or even getting on the flight to Melbourne and thinking "I have totally lost the plot, what am I doing?"

Are there any areas that you didn't learn on the course that you think would have been important for you as a full-time practitioner?

Jill: The nutrition-specific knowledge on the course was amazing; it puts you in a good position from a knowledge perspective, but in addition to that, an area I did not learn a lot about was data management. For me, it isn't exciting, and I think back to what that would have been like to teach. I have learned a lot from our data analyst at cycling. Usually, I will approach him with an idea for a data set and a vision for the output, then he can help me get to that endpoint. Data management and data analysis is important even from the aspect of ensuring that you're providing athletes with valid, true and reliable interpretations of data. Another one would be dealing with people. Dealing with stakeholders can be challenging. Learning how to manage conflict would be good. It is high-performance sport and hard conversations are part of it, so it would be good to learn more on how to manage these situations.

Recently, in my own practice, I've had a couple of difficult conversations and I thought to myself, how have I navigated that conversation, when I haven't been shown how to, or how to deal with it.

Jill: Exactly. There have certainly been circumstances where I think, 10 years ago there's no way I would have even considered this conversation with this person, in fact, even three years ago!

Where do you think the future of performance nutrition will be in five years' time?

Jill: You said it previously, but the use of technology will only increase, and also female-specific research is going to explode. It's going to be an exciting space to watch. The research on gut health will be big and potentially more testing around individualisation, which could come off the back of the gut health research. From an applied sports nutrition perspective, even in the last 5 to 10 years, more sporting programmes are embedding nutrition into the sport science department, which is exciting. It would be great to see more full-time roles for performance nutritionists in sport.

Is there a book that you've recently read which has improved your practice; now it doesn't necessarily have to be a nutrition book, it's just something that you might have read that you then put into practice?

Jill: One of the books I read last year which I found interesting was *Atomic Habits* by James Clear. I'm sure you've read it and I think probably a lot of people in the industry have. It was recommended to me from someone else, and I found it fascinating. I now receive his weekly newsletter.

I read that recently and presented elements of the book to HSBC Global, IKEA and Credit Suisse, in particular the idea of cravings and cues, leading into the cycle of developing a good habit, and then of course a bad habit. It's great when you present that to individuals that may have never considered it; the positive outcome of getting up and having a 10-minute walk in the morning before breakfast and stacking those five days in a row and suddenly, it's an extra 10,000 steps that you've never done before. I have always thought to myself it's nothing groundbreaking, you're just trying to get people to think about what they are doing.

Jill: Yeah, definitely. I think being able to apply these things into practice is the hard part. One part that registered with me was using visual cues. I make content such as putting a poster up and initially you see it every day and then one day you just don't even see it anymore. It becomes just another thing on the wall; it's in the background. I think some of those visual cues are so important and great prompts, so updating them often is important.

Are there any key principles that you try to follow every day? What things do you hold close to you that you think are important?

Jill: Exercise. I try to do some form of exercise every day, whether that is go for a run, to the gym or do yoga. I spend time building relationships with people, turning up with a smile on my face and ready to communicate (this is certainly far from perfect, but I do try... and coffee helps). Recently I have been reminding myself that spending time at a laptop is not more productive than having conversations with people, and often those documents that are produced will have minimal impact if your relationship with that person is not strong. I try to surround myself with good, positive people and understand why somebody may act the way they do, rather than jumping to conclusions. The other thing that I am currently aiming for is "progress not perfection every day"; this is a work in progress.

Recently I had anterior cruciate ligament (ACL) surgery and so I challenged myself to get through it as quick as I could. After 11 weeks from the ACL reconstruction and meniscus tear, I ran a 5K in 26 minutes. The exercise was important for both my mental and physical health. Without the garage gym that we've got at home, I would struggle. It's 45 minutes each day where I play music and take myself away.

Jill: Yeah, definitely. I did a couple of weeks of home quarantine in Australia where I was only allowed to leave the house for medical attention. It was interesting, but exercise was important. I just rotated around a few different types of exercise and created a routine. I love a routine.

Are you someone that diarises content every day?

Jill: From a work perspective 100%; I put everything in my calendar. All the tasks that need to be done go in the calendar and I dedicate time to them. Outside of work, things in my personal life are more of a mental note of what is taking place that week.

In your opinion, what do you think makes a successful performance nutritionist?

Jill: It feels funny answering this question as I am very early on in my career. However, I think one element is having that passion for excellence, passion to continuously improve, and the drive to improve your nutrition-specific knowledge. If you're not passionate, it is very obvious in high-performance sport. Consistently working hard is key; it's a tough industry to be in and with it being so popular, there's a conveyor belt of new people waiting to take your role. This was something that Professor James Morton mentioned to me recently: "The goal posts are always changing, and nothing lasts forever". Contracts in Olympic sports are often only for four years, so I think getting used to living with a level of uncertainty and that things may change (which I'm not always very good at) is key.

Eddie Hearn, from Matchroom Sport, has a podcast called "No Passion, No Point". He basically says, unless you're passionate about it, there's no point doing it. I like this because when you look at people that are successful in their sport, or in their industry, whether they're a musician or a ballet dancer, there's a core passion about what they do. I think that's a key one for many to consider.

Jill: That is interesting, and I would agree. The day you lose that spark, you're probably not going to last too much longer.

MY REFLECTIONS FROM JILL'S INTERVIEW

One thing I love about this interview is the sheer determination that Jill has shown to get where she is in her career at present. Even early on when she was told she did not have the experience to do the job that she had applied for, but was persistent and asked them to give her the chance and she would prove them wrong. Would you have the same courage?

For students who are thinking about transitioning from a MSc degree to a PhD, take a leaf out of Jill's chapter and ask people what it is like. I respect this from Jill; she sat down and asked lecturers and PhD students what it's like to study a PhD. There are too many students who progress into the next stage of their studies because they don't know what else to do but at the same time have not asked what it is like to continue with further studies!

Again, we read about a practitioner who jumped and took the chance, backed herself and expected that the net would catch her! Moving to the other side of the world to have a career takes a lot of courage and willpower and Jill should pat herself on her back with a life-changing move like that. Jill also speaks about how timing is everything and I agree with this.

Finally, I like how Jill reflects on the Olympic planning meetings which are clearly memorable for her. Sometimes it isn't the gold medal that we remember but all the behind-the-scenes planning and preparation for the long journey ahead to reach a winning performance!

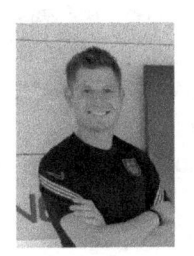

CHAPTER 8:
DR CHRIS ROSIMUS

Since 2011, Chris has worked in professional sport, starting with the England and Wales Cricket Board for nearly six years. During this period, Chris was also a performance nutritionist with the English Institute of Sport, Leicester City Football Club and Aston Villa Football Club. Recently Chris has worked as the Men's Lead Performance Nutritionist at The Football Association with England football. This is where Chris and I met and have worked together for the last four years.

Chris holds an undergraduate degree in Human Nutrition from Manchester Metropolitan University and a Master's degree in Sport and Exercise Science from Sheffield Hallam University. In 2020 Chris completed his Professional Doctorate in Sport and Exercise Science from the University of Kent.

Chris, we've had the pleasure of working with each other for the last four years, however can you provide a bit of information about your background and journey into the role you are in now?

Chris: I started out in the world of performance nutrition in 2010, when I started working with the English Institute of Sport (EIS). At that time, I was specifically working within the England Cricket team. I spent six years with EIS. I really enjoyed this period and had multiple roles. My main role was to look after the men's and women's team but also the pathway players below the senior teams. I also had a contract with England Squash as part of my EIS role. I have previously worked in para-equestrian and alongside that I was a consultant nutritionist for a six-year period which included work with Nottingham Forest Football Club and Leicester City Football Club between 2014 and 2017, and with Aston Villa Football Club. In 2017 I joined The English Football Association to lead the nutrition department across the men's and women's pathway and that's where I am now.

Your actual first involvement in nutrition was when and how many years ago?

Chris: My first proper job was 2010, but my journey into nutrition wasn't the classic route. When I left school in the late 90s, I went straight into work. My dad was a gas engineer, and I followed him into the profession. I started by working for him, but after six months, I realised this wasn't working for me. I was living away from home, spending more time messing about rather than doing the job. I vividly remember my dad making me go to the job centre and saying to me "Find a job that works for you because this isn't for you". I got a job through a friend of my dad's as an alarm engineer, which I did for six years. At that point I thought that was my job, that was my career. A career in sports nutrition was so far off my radar, I didn't even know it existed. Back in those days I just ate breakfast and lunch; I didn't really think about food as performance or health or anything like that.

Initially, my interest in nutrition was sparked through my love and passion for playing football. I still play now and in 2003, it was the sliding doors moment in my life and my career. A friend of mine at the football club where I played asked if I would help him out with coaching the junior team.

They coached kids every Saturday morning and my best mate wanted to get into coaching. He started coaching the children; he had sessions with 40 children at least twice a week and he said to me, "Come on, come and help with coaching them". At that time, I didn't want to know about it; my lifestyle on a Friday night back then was a couple of beers, play football and get on with it. The idea of getting up on a Saturday morning to coach children was not my idea of fun at the time. However, he begged me, and I said, "Right, okay I'll do it, I'll give you a hand this one time". I fell in love with it straight away and that turned into seasons of football coaching.

It was through this that I started to think about nutrition, because we used to talk to the kids about breakfast. We were training and coaching them on football, but we would also say "Right, what was your breakfast today?" We would get various answers, and back then, in the early days of the internet, my friend and I started looking at healthy breakfasts. I remember buying the Anita Bean *Sports Nutrition* book. Not because I wanted to be a sports nutritionist, but because I wanted to know what I was talking about. I started talking about nutrition to the children, and they began to take it on board and eat better. We used to train on this Astroturf pitch and next to the pitch there was a disused cricket pavilion. We used to go in it before training; it was narrow so we would clear the flooring. With all the kids in there we would deliver a mini-lecture on porridge or something similar for breakfast. We printed out information sheets on nutrition, again not because I wanted to be nutritionist, but because these children responded to the information and wanted to eat better.

Ultimately, I was delivering nutrition back then and that snowballed. When I started to do my level two football coaching badge, there was a section on nutrition for football. That really sparked my interest in nutrition and so it was around 2005 where I realised that I didn't want to be an alarm fitter for the rest of my life, and I wanted to take the steps towards a career in nutrition. I explored how to get into it and it went from there.

Good background. Who are some of your biggest mentors in your life and why have they been important to you?

Chris: There have been different people along the way. I guess there are different chunks of your life where you're immersed in different environments and there are various people that you meet along the way that guide you through it, although these people haven't stayed as a mentor all my life.

In the early days when I was coaching football, some of the coach educators I met were brilliant. They gave me a lot of confidence and it was quite inspirational to watch how they operated. There are various people that inspired me. When I started my studies and lectures at university, I remember those who took the time out to guide me. I was always asking questions as a student. When I went to university, I was a mature student at 23. I had a clear focus of where I wanted to go, so I would go and see the lecturers who I enjoyed listening to and ask them questions. They would always be a source of guidance for me throughout the period that I was studying. Then when I got into nutrition working for England Cricket, the head of physiotherapy was super. He was a great source of support because in the early days at cricket, I felt like I was fighting against the tide a little bit. I felt I was quite underqualified. Although I had my degree and my master's, I still felt underprepared for the world of nutrition. However, my mentor gave me a lot of protection and I am so thankful for that.

Additionally, my dad has got an unbelievable work ethic and that's stuck with me. His motto is "It's not right, until it's right" and I have that same approach to what I'm doing. In presentations if a font or text is not a certain way, I'm not satisfied until I feel it's right. His work ethic has 100% stuck with me.

Right now, my wife is probably my biggest mentor. She's a medic and she inspires me every day, seeing how she operates and the stories she tells me. Her work ethic and level of intelligence is brilliant. In summary, although different people have inspired me, what they have taught me has definitely remained. The things I have learnt I try and pass on to people like you.

What's been a standout moment for you in your career?

Chris: The biggest moment I'm most proud of was when I got my first full-time role as a nutritionist with England Cricket. I say this because of my previous career as an alarm engineer. I had to start again. I had no qualifications at school; I had to do a foundation year and learn basic chemistry and biology again. Overnight I went from putting cables up at a building site, to learning equations the next day in the lecture room at university. I thought to myself, I can't do this, this is absolutely beyond me. However, from reading textbooks and learning again I got through it. I remember studying English and learning how to write an essay again because I hadn't done it for so long.

So, getting on the degree programme and being surrounded by all these young students allowed me to build lots of experiences. For example, whilst I was studying, I had many internships and I sought out experiences that cost me lots of money. At the time, my five-year plan was to work with the English Institute of Sport. After America I had a job working in Abu Dhabi as a football coach and I delivered education on basic nutrition for football. I'll never forget the moment I had the interview with EIS and they rang me, and I was offered the job. The satisfaction and relief were immense and that for me is probably the biggest moment because that set me on this career path that I always wanted.

I've also been lucky with the roles that I have had. I have been fortunate to spend my career working at the national level of England Cricket, and consulting at Leicester City Football Club when they won the Premier League. As a football fan, this was an absolute dream come true. It was an unbelievable experience. Then all the way to the present day, now working at The Football Association. There are several great moments, but the biggest standout moment was actually getting my first job at England Cricket.

What do you think is the most influential factor as to why you've been successful?

Chris: The biggest factor, without a doubt, is commitment and hard work. To be committed to everything that I had set out to do. To change the role and to have a vision of where I wanted to go, and to stick to it, even when I was not guaranteed the job at the end of it, was commitment. To go through and get my degree and professional doctorate has all taken a real strong commitment and sticking to it. I would say that's been the biggest factor for me being successful with this.

I haven't waited for opportunities to come my way either; I've gone out and looked for them. When I was studying, I knew where I wanted to go, and I plotted what I would need, and I went out and looked for it. So, every opportunity that I have had, I feel like I've sorted them out myself, when I was trying to make it in the early days. Once I had obtained each role, I have been committed to each and tried to work as hard as I possibly can.

Just on that, would you say a big part of that is putting yourself out there and being open to volunteering roles?

Chris: Yes, it's essential. When I was coaching football, that was a voluntary role and within this role I started delivering nutrition, but I wasn't getting paid for that. Then whilst I was studying, I used my football coach contacts to deliver nutrition with the clubs that I was with. There was no financial backing involved in any of that. In 2009 I got a nutrition internship over in America, and this was a volunteer role. This cost me money as I had to pay to get there and spent four months in the USA. The volunteering side of it is crucial; if you can get some money for expenses, then great, but sometimes you must be prepared to do stuff for little to no money. If it's all part of where your plan is meant to take you then I would always say to myself, "It's a long-term investment in yourself".

What's been the biggest challenge of your career to date?

Chris: The biggest challenge was the feeling like I belonged in the environment that I was in. I am getting better at this now but getting over this and feeling comfortable in any new environment was a big challenge. I had come from a background that was not the classic route into sport nutrition and high-performance sport. With this, I didn't feel that I belonged in that space academically and getting comfortable with that was hard. Ultimately, I progressed through self-belief and knowing that I'm in this role for a reason, but also having the confidence and drive to keep learning and keep evolving.

With this I did the International Olympic Committee diploma and turned that into a master's. More recently I completed my professional doctorate. I've always maintained a commitment to getting the next piece of education or qualification, mainly to keep learning and to ensure I've got credibility. Credibility not necessarily from the people around me but for myself. Once I started to feel like I belonged, then I started to enjoy the work, and this was when I started to do some of what I felt was my best work. Mainly because I was so much more comfortable in my own skin.

There will be a lot of people who may not have that feeling of belonging right now due to COVID-19 implications on normal working patterns. What characteristics do you think people need to work in our industry of nutrition?

Chris: There are many characteristics. You have to be fully committed to it. You can't just come in and spend a few days here and there; this isn't enough. When you've been in a job for as long as me (11 years), you can start to grow into a role and make some good changes.

Specific to working in our environment, it's understanding that change is inevitable. I was in my role at England Cricket for five years and the turnover with coaches and staff was high; there was a lot of change. Being able to be adaptable and flex your style is important. You're going to be working with many different individuals, especially in big organisations (of several teams, each with different support networks around it) so being able to adapt your own personal style to operate in these environments is a key skill. I have also come to value and appreciate the literature that underpins our discipline. It's not just about how to flex and survive; you have got to be able to offer something and that comes with a commitment to the industry to understand more about the science, to give you more confidence as an individual and then apply this work in any environment.

If you were to advise an aspiring student coming into the industry now, what would be your recommendations considering what you know about the industry?

Chris: I reflected a lot and I had lots of good and rich life experiences before I got into my first job. These prepared me well for working in the environment and that's why I was able to survive. I volunteered a lot; I got out my comfort zone and put myself out there. I had developed well in this sense but when I look back at my studies, I wish I had better application to education and a deeper understanding of the science when I graduated. To be honest, I didn't quite have the balance right. I had good interpersonal skills and life experience, but I was lacking in the scientific knowledge, not through lack of trying; it just wasn't there. So, looking back I would try and get that balance right.

My overall advice would be to find a programme that's going to give you a blend of both. Think about how you are going to get the good underpinning science, learn something solid, but also how that is then combined with avenues into industry where you will get the opportunities to apply the knowledge. Of course, it is on you to go and look for your own opportunities, but have a think about what course at university is going to give you the best options to practise what you have been taught.

Are there any areas that you didn't learn on your course that have been important for you now you're working full time in the role that you're in?

Chris: The course I studied was a human nutrition degree. It was food based, focusing on sports nutrition with a few modules on science and performance. There weren't any behavioural change or coaching modules.

This is important because ultimately, we are nutrition coaches, but unless you are taught how to coach, how to influence and have an appreciation for behavioural science, you have to go from your own intuition or what you may have learnt yourself.

Although there is more quality science being taught in the more contemporary courses these days, the principles of teaching, coaching and behavioural change should be more engrained into programmes as this would allow students to come out with a better appreciation and more skill in these areas. This would be a welcome addition to programmes moving forward.

Where do you think the future of sports nutrition will be in five years?

Chris: It's an interesting question. When I look back I have enjoyed a decade of nutrition work. When I first got my first role in 2010, I got a job at a high level with just a degree and then I started my International Olympic Committee diploma with a view to convert it into a master's. However, in the last five years, it seems to have become a prerequisite for practitioners to hold PhDs. I used to think to myself, Christ, if I went for a job now, I'll be way off, because all I have is just a degree, going into a master's. I don't even have the PhD.

I do wonder how that trend will change. For example, now you see that a PhD seems to be the new master's and PhDs that are being combined with the rich immersive industry skills like the PhD you have completed yourself. It makes me think about the educational journey that new practitioners go on and what skills they will be equipped with. On one side are those coming through who have lots of skills and are super knowledgeable with the academic content because they specialise in an area so much over 3-4 years. However, will this therefore create a shortfall in practitioners who can operate and thrive in the elite sports setting?

As such, it would be very interesting to see how the future career paths change for our industry. I've been doing some research myself for my professional doctorate. I have been looking at all the different courses in the UK, MScs and undergraduate degree programmes, and there aren't a great deal of courses that are offering coaching science and how-to-teach principles in their programmes. One or two are doing this and seem to be incorporating this into their programmes, so it will be interesting to see what type of practitioner graduates in five years' time. Will it be a strong hybrid of both skill sets?

Yeah, I agree. If there was an MSc that incorporated the core underpinning fundamental knowledge that you need to know, combined with behavioural science and the ability to coach it well, you could argue that this could be just as valuable as someone who's got an unbelievably mechanistic PhD but an inability to coach an athlete.

Chris: I think this area is going to be interesting to see how universities will embrace the change. Is it because they want to, or does it become a core part of the programme delivery?

Is there a book that you've read recently which has improved your practice?

Chris: We have talked about this book many times; I really enjoyed the David Goggins book titled *Can't Hurt Me*. I think the lessons of hard work and commitment resonated with me. It also made me reflect and think, am I really operating to my optimal? Am I giving the most that I can give all the time or am I operating at 50% of my capacity? It's really helped me look at my own practice and think am I doing myself justice with my current output. For me that was an interesting book.

In the past, a book I was given by my mentor in my early days when I was struggling, was called *Hostage at the Table* by George Kohlrieser. It was a book about someone who was a hostage negotiator and worked as a commando in the USA. It described how he would operate in that kind of hostage situation and negotiate with various criminals. The book spoke about the process you would go through during negotiations and then how these principles may be able to be applied to your own practice. For example, people who you may struggle to work with or maybe a colleague you may struggle to influence in a certain way. It was a key book that helped me in my early days.

Are there any key principles that you try to follow every day?

Chris: I like to have routine and structure, more so now than ever in the world that we are currently operating in. From my working background when I was fitting alarms and working for my dad, a working day for me started at nine and you finished at five. In our roles we are lucky because there's flexibility, but I always try and treat each day like a working day as best I can. Some days you can do less, some days you do more, but I always try and approach my day and try and fill it the best I can. I'm a big believer in having a routine and structure that can be worked around.

Finally, with your experience and in your own view, what do you think makes a successful performance nutritionist?

Chris: From my own research, but also from my own experiences, it's individuals that can flex and adapt to any situation. This is important, because environments change, job roles change, every environment is different and there are multiple environments. If you can flex your style to work with the colleagues around you that's a huge trait of a successful practitioner, but also with the athletes that you're working with. Normally you may have 20–30 athletes; everyone will have a different style of learning and it's important you are able to adapt your style to meet the style of the athlete.

The most successful practitioners are the ones that can operate in any team structure and when it comes down to it, they can operate with any individual during a one-to-one. If you can influence someone's nutritional behaviours consistently, with 24 different players in one team, and influence them to various levels, that's the biggest thing. If you can't do that, you have got to question your impact that you are aiming to have. Therefore, being able to flex your style across any environment, and be good with your one-on-one with the athlete, in my opinion are the biggest traits that can act as a marker of success for nutritionists in the industry.

MY REFLECTIONS FROM CHRIS'S INTERVIEW

Chris has a bit of a unique journey into sports nutrition considering he was an electrician beforehand and had to go back and study basic sciences at college again! This did not stop him on his way to the top but one thing to point out is how even from the early days of studying Chris was always asking questions. Even when he felt out of place and felt underprepared, he maintained always asking questions. Personally, when I have taught at universities, it's the students that ask the questions that I always remember.

Commitment pops up again from Chris's interview and how he felt like he went out and grabbed every opportunity he could. This is a key lesson for those reading this book to think about. How often have you sat there thinking you never get the opportunities, but the real question to ask yourself is how often have you reached out to look for the opportunities?! This links nicely into how Chris volunteered as much as possible and knew that this was only ever going to be a long-term investment into his own personal growth and development.

Finally, having worked in many different environments myself from team sports to individual sports, I know how important it is to flex your style and adapt to the department that you are in. Some people do this well and others struggle with this. Spend some time thinking about when you flexed your own style well, and what was it you did to achieve this?

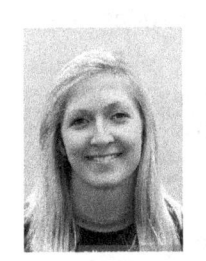

CHAPTER 9:
EMMA GARDNER

Emma currently works as the Lead Performance Nutritionist at the English Institute of Sport (EIS) working with England Men's Cricket and Great Britain Women's Hockey and has worked in elite sport for the last nine years.

Emma has an undergraduate degree in Sport and Exercise Science from the University of Birmingham and a Master's degree in Sport and Exercise Science with Psychology from Manchester Metropolitan University. Her second master's is in Sport and Exercise Nutrition from London Metropolitan University and Emma also holds the International Olympic Committee Diploma in Sports Nutrition.

Although Emma and I have never worked or studied together, I made sure I contacted Emma and networked with her. We have stayed good friends since and always enjoy a good chat about all things nutrition and improving athlete performance.

You can follow Emma on Twitter @EmGardner1

Emma, can you provide a little bit of information about who you are and what your background is?

Emma: I'm currently a performance nutritionist working for Great Britain women's hockey and England Cricket. I did my undergraduate degree in Sport and Exercise Science at the University of Birmingham. I then progressed on to a master's at Manchester Metropolitan University studying sport and exercise science again, but with a psychology branch to it. I therefore graduated with a Master's in Sport and Exercise Science with Psychology.

Following this course, I got a job working with Lucozade Sport in their sport science team and this had a nutrition focus. An aspect of the role I liked within this job was the applied nutrition aspect of teams who had Lucozade as a sponsor. Typically, we would go into clubs and provide nutrition education about the Lucozade products to the practitioners. Following this, I then applied to do an internship with the English Institute of Sport, where I applied to do the internship within sports nutrition. I was successful at getting this internship and so I then decided to study again but this time a second master's in sports nutrition. Sometimes people ask me why I have two MScs. It's not because I wanted to; it was purely because I began my career thinking I wanted to have a career in sports psychology. I then realised working in sports nutrition was where I wanted to be and so went and got the right qualifications in that area. I'm glad I did a master's in sports psychology; I think it's helped me to align the two practices together.

During my time with EIS, I graduated from a student internship into other roles which over the past 7–8 years have allowed me to work with a range of sports clubs including Northampton Saints Rugby, professional football teams alongside GB Hockey and women's rugby age groups. As I mentioned earlier, in the last few years I have been working full time with England Cricket.

What would you say your first role in nutrition was?

Emma: My interest in nutrition started when I worked with Lucozade Sport. As much as I enjoyed nutrition within my sport and exercise science degree,

I started to learn about the applied side of how you actually take the science and put that into practice for the athlete. However, my first actual role in nutrition was when I got the internship at EIS. I was working with a range of sports but mainly younger athletes who were essentially starting out in their careers, which fitted well as I was starting out as a sports nutritionist. The good thing about the internship was that I was doing it at the same time I was studying for my master's, so I could take the science and apply it immediately with the athletes. One day I'd learn about protein synthesis and then the next day I could implement this into an actionable strategy. Sometimes practitioners lack this approach because once your studies have been completed you move on to working in the applied field and might not read important literature anymore. I did the two together which in hindsight was probably a good thing for me.

I would support that comment. My experience at Widnes Vikings Rugby Club provided for by Professor Graeme Close was what you may call in at the deep end! I was in the club and now the nutritionist for 35 rugby players. Graeme said, "Go and do a good job!" I was like, "Right, here we go, what do I do?" and he was like, "Mate, you wanted this role, figure it out!"

There I was, exactly as you said, sitting in a lesson at university learning about muscle protein synthesis and then the next day educating the players about eating more protein because it was going to support their recovery. The majority of university courses are great at providing the core fundamental principles of sport nutrition but may lack the opportunity for applied experience.

Who are some of your biggest mentors in your life and why are they important for you?

Emma: Early on in my career it was Mark Ellison. Mark is the nutritionist at British Boxing. There was a slight connection with Lucozade Sport being a sponsor of British Boxing and we are both from the north of England. As a Lucozade representative, I would go into the boxing building quite often. I can remember watching Mark work a couple of times and he ignited my passion to get into the applied work with athletes. I kept thinking to myself, what a job that is, you're working in a field that you love, but you're directly working with athletes to support their performances. I chewed his ear off a million times asking if I could shadow him at work for a few days. I remember doing it a few times and doubting myself, thinking that I didn't know anything. I frantically wrote down as much as I could from the things he was saying. I remember ringing Mark when an advert for the boxing internship at the EIS came up. I rang him nervously and said, "Mark, this internship that's come up... am I appropriate for it and do you think I'm ready for it?" I remember him being brutally honest and he said, "Emma there will probably be about 500 people going for this role because it's paid but go for it!"

I rang him the day before my interview and ran a few things by him. I was successful with the interview and got the internship. Mark will always be a massive influence on me. He has a phenomenal ability to take complex information and articulate it in a way that allows him to flex his style across a range of people. He is one of the best people I've seen ever do it. I remember thinking I want to be like that. I want to be able to take information, make it meaningful to whoever is in front of me. Mark has been a big influence.

I also have a second mentor, James, who was one of my mentors at Lucozade Sport for five years before he went into the commercial side of sports nutrition, and I went into the applied side. Still now to this day, if I ever want an opinion on something from someone who's a bit more neutral, he's the person I would always call. It's been important for me to have a mentor outside of nutrition as well, who can give you a less emotional response because they are less attached to the situation.

Finally, Michael Naylor. When I started out on an internship in the EIS, I was placed with him. It's random how it works out; he was at Wasps Rugby at the time and then I got the role with Northampton Saints Rugby, so we had the rugby connection. Mike has a very different style to Mark, but he's always been an influence and we've always had a good connection through the EIS programme. He's somebody who has similarities with me in our approach to the human side of the job, understanding individuals and what is meaningful to them. I would say this is probably the biggest thing that I always take from Mike.

What has been a standout moment for you in your career to date?

Emma: There have been many memorable moments at work, but the outcome of the hockey girls winning the gold medal at their Olympics was special, the biggest prize in their sport. However, I remember the first time doing focused reflection about what made the team successful at that point in time and critiquing myself fully on it. Thinking about what I did well, what I didn't do well.

When I think about other moments in my career, honestly, they are the opposite; they are key moments or challenges. For example, when I started in cricket, nutrition was a discipline that was still in its infancy. Unlike all the previous sports I had worked in, where nutrition was already embedded, it took time to put nutrition on the map and shift the perception of how it could support performance. It wasn't straightforward, and it's taken a lot of time and a lot of effort to fully embed the discipline into the sport. Now 3½ years on, I think back and think we've done it, we have achieved it, and we've made nutrition meaningful, and we've put it on the map.

Is nutrition where you want it to be or is there still room to go?

Emma: Absolutely yeah, and it's probably been a good path now for 18 months. When you apply for a job and you get it, you're in there on day one. You almost assume that because a sport is employing a sports nutritionist, they want sports nutrition support. But sometimes, if it's not a given from the start, you must take a step back, be patient, and think about how you are going to embed your discipline.

A lesson to any young practitioner: some sports have had nutritionists and they've had experience of nutrition support, and they're ready for it. You simply take over from the last nutritionist and move it on again. Then there are other sports where you're trying to change a whole perception of a discipline and you are trying to add value and show how your support can influence performance. These are challenging roles, but they are rewarding and satisfying when you get there! There is still work to do as there always is in any sport, but we're now at a point where nutrition is accepted and supported. It's brilliant and continues to be the most rewarding role of my career to date.

Would you share one tool that you used to flip the attitude towards nutrition at England Cricket?

Emma: The number one thing was patience to get to a point where I was accepted in the environment. I had to sit back, observe and I had to build the trust and respect of the people around me first. Then with time, I was able to implement things that I knew would be quick big wins to help shape the environment. I didn't do any work with a single individual player for probably a year. I just purely did wider picture, bigger influences for environmental shifts. This allowed me to slowly manipulate their environment to get them buying into nutrition. Then I started to work with individuals.

The second thing was resilience. I could recite so many stories of times where I nearly gave up. However, I said to myself, "If anyone's going to change this, I'm going to do it!"

Nice and honest reflections. What do you think has been the most influential factor as to why you have been successful to date?

Emma: Relationships. Without a shadow of doubt relationships with people, nothing to do with nutrition at all. I can't stress that enough. Every environment that you work in, it's about understanding people, understanding the environment. I hate using the culture label, but understanding the culture, understanding key influences, and trying to align people to the bigger picture of what you're trying to achieve. If I look through any of the sports I've worked in, and hopefully we have had some successes, each time it came down to people understanding and having the respect for the discipline. People talk about what it takes to win; they have this idea of what this looks like, but the habits and behaviours of the sport need to align to this vision. That's the key to success, matching the two and having the relationships to get people on board to align to those goals.

I have spoken to people before about the comment of "You just have to respect the people you work with; you don't have to like them; you don't have to get on with them". I really question this. I'm not saying you must be best friends with people, but trust me, you must find a common ground with people and have a good enough relationship in the first place, to then build the respect and the trust. If you can build that and you can be accepted in the environment, you've got a greater chance of success than just somebody respecting you. I hope if somebody asked what I was like at my job, I would like to think that they would say I have solid relationships with people, there is a mutual trust, and there is respect. Hopefully people know I'm trying to build the relationships for the right reasons, and they know I'm doing it because I care about the outcome of where we're going, and I am trying to help them.

This reminds me of when I interviewed Dr Daniel Martin about his challenges in the jockey world, the perceptions of nutrition and how it should be implemented. One of Daniel's take-home messages, which you've alluded to, is just being a good person. There's a lot to be said about just being a good person in an organisation.

Emma: Yeah, 100%. Being a good person but also being firm and fair. Having good relationships is key, however when I feel strongly about something, I will speak up. People know I'd be quite relaxed about things and let things slide, but if there are critical things that I see are valuable and I feel strongly about, I would raise that. I think it's also important that you don't bow down at the point of challenge. You must remember why you're there. You are there to change things, influence and help them to win. The best practitioners do both: they are a good person, they are trustworthy and reliable, but they also create change, whilst not forgetting performance.

What has been the biggest challenge of your career to date?

Emma: I remember being selected to work for Team GB for the Rio Olympic Games; it was the steepest and biggest learning curve of my life for a period of six weeks. I got there and the food was terrible; I was a punchbag for 15 different teams, for their biggest event of their life, trying to desperately run around and figure out how I was going to make the food better. That was by far and away the biggest short-term challenge that I have ever faced.

The second one in recent years has been implementing nutrition as a discipline that is valued in cricket. Without a doubt they have been the two biggest challenges of my career. It's funny because I sometimes think if I had experienced those two experiences earlier on in my career, would I have survived them? That sounds quite dramatic but honestly, I don't think I would have done, I don't think I would have been resilient enough. I think it was probably the good experiences and the more subtle challenges that have built me up to be able to go on and deal with the more recent tougher difficulties.

There are elements of resilience I have felt too. Losing my dad a couple of years ago, the resilience that I found off the back of that was huge. For example, when I was faced with situations at work, the younger me would have got emotionally heated about the situation. Whereas the reality of losing a parent, it rocks your world, and you put everything into perspective a lot more. Now I look at situations and I rarely get emotional about it; it doesn't bother me. However, five years ago I would have had an argument with the person who said that comment.

What characteristics do you think practitioners need to work in nutrition?

Emma: When people ask that, I always think about who I see as a good practitioner and why I think that about them. Good practitioners have a great ability to communicate, as simple as that. When you have a call with some people you just chat away, and you are at ease straight away with the conversation. They have an ability to communicate in a way which draws people in and a genuine ability to listen. You know that some of the best practitioners have listened because when you pick up the phone to them, they remember information that you talked about ages ago. It might be a minor detail but it's critical because it shows that you care, and are interested in the other person.

I think another one is an ability to flex your approach. We graduate thinking each athlete is the same and they are a clone of one another. The best practitioners are the ones who can identify the different requirements of the athletes. For example, how you work with an athlete who has been to three Olympic Games will be different to an athlete who may be attending their first professional match. How you work with an athlete who is worried and needs your reassurance will be different from one who loves the science and wants to know the evidence from the latest journal article.

The best practitioners can get their message across and change a person's habits and behaviours based on the ability to flex their communication style. The last one is the ability to deliver what is needed, versus what you think they need. Everybody wants to go in and deliver a nitrate strategy because it's cool, or a menthol strategy because that's the latest thing to do. The reality is, I have worked with England Cricket for three years and we didn't go anywhere near that for the first two and a half years. Initially, we have been getting them to focus on eating the right breakfast! I get phone calls all the time; people ask what I am doing with a cool new strategy and I say, "Absolutely nothing". I don't know anything about it because that's not what they need at present. Right now, they need basic information and focus because that's what's going to make the biggest difference to their performance and their potential success.

I find myself getting irritated when I see other practitioners delivering completely the wrong thing; sometimes they deliver the new thing because they think that's what they need, but it's not. If you listen and observe properly, you'll get your biggest bang for your buck if you just deliver one very basic strategy.

If I reflect on my first year at England football, my colleague and I did nothing apart from observe the environment. At that time, players and staff were not ready for in-depth nutritional support with research embedded. I had recently finished my PhD conducting the world's first energy expenditure study in professional rugby and taking blood samples in changing rooms during live rugby games to assess muscle inflammation. I remember my colleague said to me, "England football is five years away from that". What we've got to do at the moment is observe and see where the quick wins are and what we need to work on to have the biggest impact. Exactly as you've said, the first thing that we worked on was the menu that

is provided at base camp. This process involved building relationships and working with the hotel chefs. Even more recently, working with the senior women players and the pathway players, naturally there are players that have a good nutrition knowledge, but there are players who still under-fuel. Therefore, it is important to educate them on the importance of increasing fuel each day. Sometimes going back to the basics can be impactful.

Emma: Absolutely. Sometimes, there's a pressure to do something amazing. I sit on calls with my colleagues in the EIS and hear what they are doing, and I think I am the worst nutritionist here; I don't even know anything about that. I also think wow if I worked in that sport, I'd be lost because I wouldn't be able to manage that. But you've got to work with what's in front of you; that's going to get you more success.

What would be your biggest recommendation to your younger self or to aspiring students entering the industry now?

Emma: To think and map out what you need to do in your role to be successful. I love asking junior practitioners this because sometimes the response is "I'll do a presentation on carbohydrate". I say to them how rare it can be to do this in your first year. I would recommend gaining experience and speaking to athletes. I remember my mentor advising me to do fake interviews with an athlete. It was terrifying because I had the knowledge of nutrition, but as soon as I sat with somebody, I was thinking how do I communicate this information, or get the information from them that I need to help them out?

It's quite hard today for anybody coming into the industry. We say how important it is to get experience, but even just chatting with a nutritionist who's been in the environment can help, as you can see if your perception matches to what they tell you. This can be very helpful as every environment will be different.

Also, think about other skills which are required day to day and try your best to get experience with that. For example, I wish I spent more time with chefs before I started as a nutritionist. I had never spoken to a chef in my life before this job. Fortunately, I do have a love of food myself, so I knew quite a bit about it. One of my first meetings was with a chef and I went to the meeting with some amazing ideas, and they asked me if I had ever worked in the kitchen trying to cook for 80 people before. Building relationships with chefs and thinking about what it is like on the kitchen floor was one of my biggest lessons.

Be patient and accept that you must earn your stripes. You have to take the time and the hours of hard work, the unpaid hours and the not very nice parts of the job (i.e. washing protein shakers). I vividly remember my degree dissertation. I was stood at Birmingham New Street train station, at 5am, three days a week, clicking people up and down who took the stairs versus who took an escalator. I did that for three months. I thought why am I doing this, what am I doing this for, how does this even relate? However, getting up every day at 5am, standing in the cold clicking people, I became patient and resilient. I knew this would contribute to me becoming a better person down the line.

Are there any areas that you did not cover during your degree courses that have been important for you now that you are working full time?

Emma: There need to be additions to courses to prepare practitioners for the applied sport setting. Areas that cover things like menu planning, writing catering guidelines, performing real-life consultations, and practising how you speak to athletes. One thing I do now as part of my interview process for jobs is to ask the interviewee to speak with the chef. It's a huge part of the job role, so I want them to pretend that they are now speaking with the chef and working with the chef to compromise about certain items on the menu. Then there are other aspects of our job that we do, for example how do you sit with the head coach and try and sell to him or her how your nutrition strategy is going to support their players, how do you go about scheduling in what you're going to do on the camp. All the bits of our job that you don't get taught on an academic course. I think this is what is missed.

I think it's important that moving forward this is addressed because this is why new graduates take so much longer to get up to speed. They don't have experience of those core day-to-day skills. For example, how many times do we talk about PGC-1 α versus the number of times we talk about a menu? Yet we never talk about menus when we're studying on a course. It's something that needs to be looked into, whether it is SENr courses that offer it on the course or extra sessions that can be taken. Essentially, it's these key areas that young practitioners are trying to develop.

Where do you think the future of nutrition will be in the next five years?

Emma: I think there will be a mixture of things. One of my goals for the industry is to never remove the human aspect of what we do. You know I talked around the part of being the person that you are and the relationships that you have. I think technologies are advancing all the time. For example, I think the whole gut microbiome world could be the future. Nutrition being tailored to an individual's gut microbiome.

For example, I can foresee in the future that you'll give a small stool sample, and we will base nutritional dietary guidance around a person's microbiome. There may be further development in the ultrasound technique, or non-invasive measures for assessing muscle glycogen. I think this area will advance.

However, when I look ahead in five years' time, I still think that we will have practitioners on the ground; I don't think we'll ever remove that. I know there's a fear that there will be applications that can write a meal plan for somebody by inputting a few variables and then you don't need a nutritionist to do that for you, but I still don't think you can take away the fact that we are ultimately trying to change a person's way of working and behaviours to achieve something. I think it will be two-fold. I think nutrition will advance, but there will always be a place for us because of the sheer human aspect of our job and every person is different. Therefore, I think we'll have more information to inform our strategies moving forward but I think there will always be nutrition practitioners hopefully on the ground delivering what we do best.

Is there a book you have recently read which has improved your practice?

Emma: I often read books outside of nutrition around different subjects. I recently read a book recommended by Ben Rosenblatt called *The Body Keeps the Score* (Bessel van der Kolk) which is essentially about when people have been through trauma, and how you get physiological changes based on traumatic events that have happened. It's a fascinating book about the human body and how your body adapts to certain situations.

Another fascinating one I recently read is called *The Power of Habit* (Charles Duhigg) which is very good and around how you change a person's habitual habit loops. This is applicable to our job because when you have athletes that essentially display certain behaviours that you want to manipulate, it can be a challenge to change them. It's key to remember there's a stimulus and there's an outcome. The outcome is the habit that you see, so it's important to think about how you can change the stimulus or change the routine. I think that's a critical area for practitioners to consider.

My last one links to psychology, and I know lots of people are talking about the Capability, Opportunity and Motivation Behaviour (COM-B) model (https://www.qeios.com/read/WW04E6.2) at the minute, but the closest person I've always worked with aside from strength and conditioning has always been the psychologist. In hockey, I deliver 90% of my work aligned to the psychologist, often in the room together with the athletes, because I like them to understand that the relationship with food is impacted by what and how they are thinking and feeling. I'm a massive believer in that and I like reading around psychology and understanding people and why people make the choices that they do. A lot of my reading will often be around this area.

Are there any key principles that you try to follow every day?

Emma: One thing that I am trying to work on is having respect for every person. If someone asks you for something, try not to promise something that you can't deliver on. That's a principle that I try to live by; it's not something I do every single day, but I try to commit to what I'm asked to do. My continued work is linked to communication, given I work with large teams. I need to make sure that I keep on top of communication with people and not saying I will deliver something and then not delivering it. If I can't do something for someone, rather than just fluff it, just say I can't do it. I try to live a little bit like this because with the nature of our jobs, especially in the busy world that we work in, you can quite easily fall into the trap of promising things, and you can't deliver and then that brings you down as a practitioner.

Another area is not forgetting how lucky we are to do what we do. There can be days where you think this is hard and this isn't fun. However, the reality is we are so privileged to do what we do; we have amazing jobs working with athletes to achieve their goals and I try to remind myself regularly that there are so many young practitioners trying to get jobs in our industry. We can lose sight of what we do every day. The reality is we work with lots of extremely talented and like-minded people who are trying to achieve the same goals. I try to live by that a little bit each day rather than have a routine. I try to remind myself that when it's hard at least we're doing something that we love.

What makes a successful performance nutritionist?

Emma: Without a doubt a good underpinning of knowledge; you can't ever get away from that. You don't have to be experts in everything, and I like practitioners who come on calls and admit that they don't know the answer to something. This is honesty, rather than trying to bluff that they know it. What I love about our network is the fact that there is always somebody who does have the experience. You can pick up the phone and you can find out the answer. I think that is important for any practitioner, no matter what stage of their career they are at. A good practitioner has good knowledge, but also is aware of their limitations, for example knowing what they can and can't deliver. Without a shadow of doubt delivering what's needed, not what they think is needed. This is critical to a good nutritionist.

Finally, the softer traits of having good communication, being a genuine listener and a bigger picture person who can see the long game and doesn't lose sight of what they're trying to achieve, whilst also understanding performance. I have sometimes sat with nutritionists where I have probed and asked if they fully understand what they are trying to do from a performance perspective. If you fully understand performance, then you can align to other disciplines well. If you don't fully understand what the sport entails or what you're physically trying to achieve, you're never going to be able to fulfil the capacity of your role. If you don't know that, you need to find out and then you'll find you get genuine alignment. Therefore, the last trait is an ability to genuinely align with other practitioners to influence performance.

MY REFLECTIONS FROM EMMA'S INTERVIEW

A standout part of this interview is when Emma talks about how you almost assume that because a sport is employing a sports nutritionist, they want sports nutrition support and her lesson to any young practitioner: "There are some sports that have had nutritionists and they've had experience of nutrition support, they're ready for it. You just take over from the last nutritionist and move it on again. There are other sports where you're trying to change a whole perception of a discipline and you are trying to add value and show how your support can influence performance." I have experienced this myself and it certainly takes a lot of work and determination, but when you succeed it is very satisfying.

I also agree with Emma's advice about being patient and the importance of observing first. This was something that I personally did at the FA with England football. Although it takes time to sit back and make notes, it was worth it in the end as it allowed me to really focus on what needed to be done first and create the big wins quickly.

Finally, Emma provides a nice comment on how this is an amazing industry to be working in. Yes, there are some weeks where it is difficult and the workload is heavy (like any industry), however we can genuinely impact elite athletes' performance with the knowledge and advice we are providing to them.

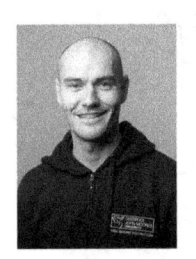

CHAPTER 10:
PROFESSOR JAMES MORTON

James is a Professor of Exercise Metabolism at Liverpool John Moores University (LJMU), where he has authored over 170 research publications related to exercise metabolism, physiology and nutrition. In addition to academia, James has also worked in a number of performance support related roles across both high-performance sport and industry. From 2010–2015, he was the performance nutritionist to Liverpool Football Club before taking up the position of Nutrition and Physical Performance Lead for Team Sky between 2015 and 2019. In this role, he was responsible for the performance nutrition strategy for five consecutive Tour de France wins. James is also the Director of Performance Solutions for Science in Sport (SiS) where he leads the Performance Solutions programme that encompasses the strategic delivery of bespoke performance solutions and innovation for SiS and their elite partners (e.g. the Ineos Grenadiers, Milwaukee Bucks and the FA women's teams). He also sits on the Technical Steering Panel for the English Institute of Sport and is a High-Performance Mentor for the FA Premier League.

I first met James when he taught me as an undergraduate student on my own sport and exercise degree at LJMU. James was one of the reasons I wanted to stay at LJMU and continue my PhD studies and I was fortunate enough to have him as a supervisor on my PhD. Through my nine-year academic journey at LJMU, I can call James a close friend and a good colleague, having co-authored multiple publications with him.

You can follow James on Twitter @JamesyMorton

Could you give an insight into who you are and what your background is?

James: I'm originally from Belfast and moved over to Liverpool when I was 18 to study a sport science degree. From the outset, I absolutely loved it in Liverpool and have been here ever since. I finished my undergraduate degree in 2003 and then progressed on to my PhD between 2003 and 2006. I then joined the academic world, so to speak, and progressed up towards professorship in 2018. Besides academic work I have also worked in elite sport with athletes from team sports, endurance sports and weight-restricted sports.

How and when did you first get involved in nutrition?

James: I've always been interested in sport, exercise, and fitness from a young age and as a teenager I was always experimenting with my own health and fitness. In doing so I would play about with different types of training programmes and so fitness and sport science always interested me. Then, during my sport science undergraduate degree, I was exposed to many topics and the one that jumped out for me was exercise physiology and metabolism.

I absolutely loved it; I couldn't get enough of it. I loved the reading side, being in the labs and seeing it all come together in practice. I was fortunate enough to publish my BSc dissertation on hypoxic training and it was then that I really developed a passion for research. In those days, you didn't necessarily need to do an MSc so I went straight to a PhD. It was then that we started taking muscle biopsies and so I started to really understand muscle physiology. However, I still didn't consider nutrition as an applied outcome of exercise metabolism. Back when I was studying, I'd always wanted to be a fitness coach because that was the applied element of physiology. At that time I hadn't really linked that a sports nutritionist was the applied outcome of someone who is interested in metabolism.

Then when I did my post-doctoral studies, I conducted an eight-week training study where we were studying how exercise training affected heat shock proteins' (or HSPs') expression in muscle. Essentially, I ran a training study looking at how carbohydrate availability could potentially upregulate HSP expression. What we discovered in that study was that carbohydrate availability didn't actually affect HSPs, but it did affect some of the mitochondrial enzymes that typically increase in response to endurance training.

It blew my mind. We had three groups of people performing the same training sessions but the group that restricted carbohydrate got the better training response in terms of some of those mitochondrial enzyme adaptations.

This is when I started to realise that nutrition was about more than just performance on match day or race day. Rather, I began to appreciate that what you eat before, during and after every single training session can completely change how your muscle adapts to exercise. From that point on, I really started developing an applied research interest in nutrition, whilst still underpinned by basic human metabolism and physiology. However, now my questions were more aligned to a nutritional intervention as opposed to a training intervention where I had previously been interested in changing the training stimulus e.g. intensity, duration, work-rest ratio etc.

It was around this time when I was 25 years old that I went into one of the local boxing clubs in Liverpool to start boxing as a hobby. Some of the guys at the boxing club found out what I did for a job, and so I began helping some of the amateurs in relation to making weight for their contests. This was all voluntary work for a few years with some of the amateurs and professionals who were living in Liverpool. On reflection, it is during this time where I learnt the basis of my trade. I made a lot of mistakes that you need to make in order to learn. I learnt basic work placement skills, if you like, and this really provided the foundation to then go on and work in professional sport in the years to follow. I still keep in touch with many of those lads and some went on to become really good friends.

Who are your mentors and why they have been important in your life?

James: Over and above work, and I think like you, James, my dad was my biggest mentor and still is. Unfortunately, my dad was killed in a car crash during my PhD but I am unbelievably thankful that I had him in my life for 22 years. I think your parents, and in particular your dad, teaches you what is right and what is wrong, how to do the right things, moulds your values, your character, what things matter to you and so on. Materialistic things don't matter to me. He taught me not to be jealous of people and count your blessings every single day. These character traits have been taught by my dad. As a young boy, I would often see my dad kneeling beside his bed every morning and night. I once asked him what he was doing and he responded by saying he was thanking God for me, my two sisters and my mum. What an example to set to a young boy.

Moving into the work environment, one of the biggest mentors I have had is Professor Steve Peters who is a clinical psychiatrist but who has worked in both clinical practice and elite sport. He helped me understand who I really am as a person, why I think the way I do and how some of my life experiences have shaped how I think. The second was Sir Dave Brailsford. Dave taught me everything about true high performance, culture, coaching and leadership. It is no exaggeration to say that the five years that I spent with Dave changed me as a person; it challenged me professionally and personally and made me better. I think anyone who spends time in Dave's company will emerge a more accomplished thinker.

At that time of your career, was the mentorship with Dave something that you actively pursued? For example, you saw the opportunity with Dave, and you didn't want to pass on this or was it just part of being in that environment at Team Sky?

James: When I joined Team Sky back in 2015, I had worked at Liverpool Football Club for five years as the sports nutritionist, but I had probably gone stale. Looking back, I didn't really understand "performance" and like many younger practitioners, I think I was just providing a service to a group of athletes. I wasn't really impacting their performance. The opportunity came to work at Team Sky and that was a great opportunity for me for two reasons. One, because carbohydrate metabolism was my research passion and there's no better place in the world to study carbohydrate metabolism than with some of the best endurance cyclists in the world. Secondly, the opportunity to work with Dave was one of the big attractions because Dave is one of the best leaders in global sport, one of the biggest and most recognised high-performance thinkers. I wanted to go and learn everything that I could from Dave based on his experiences in sport. I actively sought that out and Dave took me under his wing and mentored me through those five years to teach all things performance, culture, coaching and leadership.

Are Dave and Steve still your mentors now?

James: Definitely. I speak to them frequently; we are still in contact, and they are both at the end of the phone. If I ever have any questions, want a second opinion, feedback, or want to be challenged, then I would pick up the phone no problem. When you meet people who can improve you, it is important to keep them close and keep learning from them.

What would you say has been the biggest standout in your career to date?

James: Like many people would probably say, I guess there are too many moments to have a standout. For me, it's all been about the journey and there have been many moments along the way that have taught me something. A key thing to do is to bring that journey into different chapters. For example, and as you will know, the PhD is an incredible journey because you're getting paid to study something that you absolutely love. I was taking biopsies for the first time, understanding muscle metabolism, and it was an unbelievable time. I then completed my post-doctoral training and developed a passion for nutrition. More recently, building the research team at LJMU with Graeme Close (one of my closest friends) over the last 10 years, and especially in those first five years was (and still is) a fantastic journey. Our team went from just Graeme and I sharing an office to having a room full of over 30 PhD students, many of whom are now good friends like yourself. Whilst their academic journey has been one thing, it is the lifelong friendships and the laughs and memories we have had along the way which really do mean the most to me.

Then of course there is the sports side of things, which is all the different athletes and sports that I have worked with. This includes the boxers and combat sports athletes, my time with Liverpool Football Club and the Team Sky chapter. Now, I'm spending more time working in industry with Science in Sport, learning a whole host of commercial and business skills which is challenging me in a completely different way. So, rather than standout moments, I think my career is a series of chapters that have all taught me something new.

What I would say, though, is that my rate of personal growth was probably highest during the Team Sky chapter and that was because it was such a high-performing team, an incredibly demanding team, with high expectations and ambitions. It was an unbelievable culture to be around. At that time, I believe Team Sky were one of the most high-performing and consistently performing teams in world sport. Reflecting on time at Team Sky, two of the highlights are probably from 2018.

Winning the Giro d'Italia with Chris Froome in May and then winning the Tour de France with Geraint Thomas in July is a period of my life that will always stay with me. They were two athletes that I got close to in the previous three or four years. I know they've spoken publicly about the impact that I have made in their journeys and those wins in particular. Whilst we don't do it for public recognition, when you know that you have made a genuine meaningful difference to people and their performance, it's incredibly satisfying.

But again, to go back to what I'm most proud of, it's what we have done at Liverpool John Moores University and the people that we've created. I can think of many different people working in academia and sport who have all developed through the LJMU system. I'm sure that when both Graeme and I look back on our career in years to come, what we'll be most proud of, is the people that we've helped to produce.

It's been nice to interview other practitioners for this book, many of whom have been part of LJMU. When I have asked them who's the mentor, who is the person that they hold close to their development and career, it is yours and Graeme Close's names that crop up time and time again.

James: That's fantastic to hear, James, because again, whilst we don't do it for that recognition, I am especially proud of the fact that such people value their time at LJMU. I truly believe that LJMU is one of the most special institutes in the world. I should have in fact mentioned earlier, that the late Professor Tom Reilly was also an inspiration and mentor to me. Tom built sport science at LJMU to what it is today and I will be forever grateful that I had the privilege to work with Tom. I often stop to look at the Tom Reilly Building when I come to work each day to just have a moment of respect for what Tom did for our discipline. I am passionate about keeping Tom's legacy alive.

You might not like the way that I frame this next question because I know how your brain thinks, but what do you think has been one of the most influential factors as to why in your career you've been successful today?

James: You're probably right. I often get uncomfortable when people say I'm successful. What I can say, without doubt, is that I truly love what I do as a job. It is not a job for me, it's a passion. There are still days when I wake up and I can't believe that I'm actually getting paid to study exercise. When you look at other people around the world doing arduous jobs that they don't get excited about, I think it's a real shame. This is the perfect job for me; there's no better job for me because I truly have found my passion and passion is the basis of any perceived success.

I'm sure you've heard it many times, but I think on top of that passion, you need a real work ethic. I would say that maybe one of the reasons why people may perceive me to be successful is that I have a work ethic that might be a lot bigger than others. People often say to me that I can soak up more pressure and I can apparently do more tasks or tolerate more load than others. I will admit, though, that sometimes this has been to my detriment because I have worked too much, and I have lost balance at times. I am getting better at achieving balance as I get older.

Aside from both passion and ethic, I personally would say that one of the things I have worked hardest on over the years is communication. I've always strived to be the best communicator I can be, whether that's written or verbal or in scenarios such as giving a conference presentation, delivering a small group session, or if it's a one-to-one conversation. I have always believed that the most skilled people in life are the ones that really know how to listen, then understand and then communicate. Again, both Steve Peters and Dave Brailsford are absolute masters at that craft. As I said, it's probably the one thing that I have worked hardest at, and still do on a daily basis.

What has been the biggest challenge in your career to date?

James: Probably the biggest challenge I would say is suffering the loss of both parents; my dad died in a car accident when I was 22 and then my mum died of cancer when I was 29. Looking back, I didn't realise how it affected me at the time and I don't think I really dealt with it. What I did do was block it out and threw myself into work. I was so busy with work, sometimes fulfilling two full-time jobs at the same time. I didn't have time to think about what happened. I loved the roles that I was doing so much that I didn't realise that I wasn't dealing with the loss. I was so busy and enjoying what I was doing. However, moving forward several years, especially in the last three or four years, I've realised that I didn't deal with it, and I've had to go back and deal with it. I've now accepted that I'll always be a workaholic. That's why I'm the person that I am, partly because it's my passion, partly because of my ambition and my desire to always improve and achieve. That's just who I am and it's the way I'm made. However, as I am getting older, I'm starting to get more balance in life, and I have realised how important balance really is for overall happiness and longevity in your career. Every one of us will have to deal with grief at some point in their life. When it happened to me, I felt like the loneliest person in the world and didn't really open up or process what had actually happened. It was like my connection to Belfast had disappeared. Thankfully, as I approach 40, I believe I have come out the other side and have worked hard in the last few years to finally move on.

Just going back to Professor Steve Peters and when you worked with him to find out who you truly were, did Steve have to go back and tap into the period where the loss of your parents occurred as a younger man?

James: Yes, we did a lot of stuff on that, though I guess one of the most simple exercises that Steve gets us to do is to ask, what type of person would you like to be? I would write all those things down and eventually you realise that this is the person that you really are. However, things happen to you in your life day to day, week to week, month to month, year to year that prevent you from being that person. Ultimately, I realised that the type of person I wanted to be was someone who had balance, who worked hard, who had fun, who helped others, who enjoyed family and friendship and essentially revolved around being a good dad and setting good examples. When I realised that that was the person I wanted to be but that I was not always delivering on it because I was getting sidetracked with many other things, I knew I had to correct it.

Nowadays, I come back to these things on a daily basis. Am I being a good role model and teaching my children correctly, am I doing the right things for people around me? It's almost a form of recalibration. It allows you to stop and think. You don't really need to go and do that extra bit of work right now; instead go out and spend time with your family. You don't really need to write that paper today; you can do it tomorrow. I had created many false deadlines in my life but the most important deadline of all is raising children appropriately. So... it's fair to say that Steve had a big impact on me and helping me understand balance and "balance" for me now is what truly defines success.

What characteristics do you think people need to work in performance nutrition or high-performance sport?

James: Let's deal with performance nutrition to start with. First, you must understand how nutrition affects performance. Whilst it sounds obvious, I'm not sure many people really grasp this. To understand how nutrition affects performance, the first step is understanding human metabolism and physiology. The next step is to then understand how nutrient availability modulates metabolism and physiology. Then you can put the two together. This is what a good performance nutritionist should be doing: understanding how nutrition impacts performance and doing so in two parts. One, understanding human metabolism and then secondly understanding determinants of performance. By putting them together you come up with the practical solution for the athlete to implement. Having a strong theoretical basis of science first and then second, developing practical performance solutions.

In terms of characteristics, someone who has a scientific type of mindset, who can think logically, think clearly, break down problems and then arrive at a simple solution. Considering performance nutrition is a scientific-based discipline, you need to have a logical way of thinking. As I mentioned earlier, like in all professions where you deal with people, communication is key. That's probably one of the most critical skills that we all need to have, the ability to communicate, certainly for working in high-performance sport.

There are also wider attributes which are the obvious ones. You must be resilient, have a good work ethic, be emotionally intelligent, be willing to adapt, be willing to change, be willing to accept that what made you win two years ago might not make you win today. You must be willing to change, willing to receive feedback and act on that feedback that you receive from others. These are general skills for the person who wants to work in high-performance sport.

One thing I would say, though, is anyone who works in sports and sport science, the biggest thing that underpins it for me, is you must be passionate about exercise to start with. You must love fitness, you must love health, you must love nutrition as a person yourself. Otherwise, I don't believe you can work in that environment. You must be able to talk the language that athletes talk; you have got to know the sport, know the stories. Ideally you need to be immersed in the sport. Sport must be a true part of you and always will be if you truly want to make a difference when you work in sport.

I know you're into your podcasts now and Eddie Hearn, from Matchroom Sport, has his own podcast called "No Passion, No Point". This conversation reminds me of that!

What would be your biggest recommendation to your younger self or to aspiring students entering the industry now?

James: I've been incredibly lucky with the journey that I have been on and the people that I have been around at different times. That's where I would start. I would surround yourself with excellent mentors from the beginning of your journey; that is my number one tip. We can only go so far ourselves; at some point you need someone to guide you, to encourage you, but also challenge you and to ask tough questions of yourself, put pressure onto yourself, make you uncomfortable. The reality is, James, in every mistake that we make, someone else has made it before us, so why wouldn't you want to learn from someone who has made your mistakes and been on the same journey that you have? You know me well enough now; I've got books at home full of reflections and learnings of what other people have taught me. I'm always thinking about the kind of things I can learn from this person or from that person.

I think mentors are critical because they ask the right questions of you at the right time and for me that's what leadership is. You need someone to "ask" the right questions of you, not "telling" you what to do. Telling doesn't work; good coaching and leadership is asking you the right questions at the right time in your life when you're ready to be asked that question. If you can find someone to do that, then they are worth their weight in gold.

The second thing I would say is to read constantly and be unbelievably curious about the literature. It still amazes me now how many younger practitioners or sports scientists don't read as much as they should. More alarming, they're not curious, they've got no questions. They're not formulating any new research questions, they're not wondering about any topics that they see in their practice, there's no curiosity. A lack of curiosity will kill your career.

Finally, take time to enjoy things a lot more and not concentrate or worry about the outcome. What I've realised is that there is no clear end; there's never an end to what we do. As your career progresses, you go and get a PhD and think things will be happier or calm down; when I finish my post-doctoral training things will be alright, when I get my professorship, everything will be alright. If we win this race everything will be alright. The problem is, there is no end and I think once you realise that and accept that there's never an end it will allow you to enjoy things more.

I wish during my career I had taken some time to slow down a bit and stop and look around and go "wow", how good is this, what an enjoyable journey, how exciting is this, just take some time to really reflect and enjoy it as opposed to constantly going 1000 miles an hour towards a destination. A few years ago I went for a job interview (which I never got!) and the panel member asked me what the last bit of feedback was I had received from someone. It was actually along the lines of "Why don't you slow down for a year or a two". The panel member knew me personally and joked they agreed with that. At that time, however, I responded with "Yeah, but that doesn't wash with me". A few years later, I feel like I probably have slowed down a bit. I've worked hard on balance and I genuinely feel happier than ever.

Simon Sinek talks about the infinite purpose or the infinite game. For example, a game of football has a clear start, middle and end. Once the full-time whistle has been blown, the game is finished. However, in business and in life there's no start, middle and end. If life is like an infinite game, then you need to ask yourself the question: what is your infinite purpose in life? The infinite purpose in your world was not necessarily to get the professorship because once you achieved that then this stage was finished, but it's a greater meaning than that to you as an individual. It's almost like trying to find your passion in life; once you find your infinite purpose in life if you're abiding by that every single day then you will be happy!

Are there any areas that you didn't learn on your sport science course that you think would have been important for you as a full-time practitioner?

James: One thing I wish I would have learned earlier in my career would have been coaching and leadership skills, which is slightly different from behaviour change. People are using the term behaviour change now because it's contemporary and exciting. However, I'm talking about real fundamental coaching and leadership which is a discipline in its own right and has been formally studied for centuries. Having said that, I'm not sure that I would have been ready years ago, as an 18- to 25-year-old. To learn coaching and leadership would have been difficult at that age. Early on in my career, I was spending more time learning the technical knowledge that I needed to learn. It was only really when I became more experienced in my career, and I saw expert coaches and expert leaders at work, that I truly appreciated the science and art of leadership and coaching. Maybe you can't learn that at a younger age, however you can certainly be made more aware of it. I now try and bring that into my teaching that I do. For example, it could be more lectures on leadership philosophy and what makes a good leader and studying leaders and cultures. A good question to think about is, what does it mean to be a coach or to teach? What does it mean to be a good teacher? One of the most famous coaches of all time, Bill Walsh, frequently said something along the lines of teaching being our top priority. At the end of the day, that's all we're doing in sport science. We are in the coaching profession. Why shouldn't we be skilled in coaching? I'd love to be an expert coach and an expert leader, someone who could really inspire and help others. As I have become more experienced, I've realised life is about people and that the workplace is about people management; that's part of everything we do. I wish someone had told me that at an earlier part of my career.

Where do you think the future of performance nutrition will be in five years' time?

James: I think we'll see the rise of personalised nutrition in both health and performance. What I mean by that is whilst there are many generic principles that we could all adhere to, all these principles need to be individualised to that person for what will make a difference to them. Personalised nutrition for me doesn't necessarily mean magical genetic testing. Personalised nutrition is personalising the solution for what you need at this moment in time, for your sport, for your performance priority etc. We're starting to see this more and more with nutritional periodisation but nutritional personalisation will be the new term. So... I think we'll see the rise of the term "personalised nutrition" but the application of it really comes back to that individualisation of nutritional solutions.

Having said that, I think there is a lot more opportunity to apply what we already know. I would like to see more nutritionists in the future become better practitioners at delivering what we already know should be delivered. Let's take a simple example of the day before a race or the day before a match. Athletes still don't eat enough fuel and yet we have known this for 50 years. This is just one simple example of a whole broader array of topics where we're applying less than 10% of what we know. We need to become better at applying what we already know. The science of delivery will improve at a rapid rate.

Is there a book that you've recently read which has improved your practice?

James: There are loads of books. I love reading and am constantly reading and re-reading many books. Of three authors who have had a big impact on me, one was Bill Walsh's *The Score Takes Care of Itself*. Walsh of course is the famous NFL coach who transformed the San Francisco 49ers. He did this through a continuous improvement approach.

I love Dale Carnegie's book on *How to Win Friends and Influence People*. There is so much in that book on people management, relationships and communication. Again, if we applied 5% of the content of that book to every conversation, the world would be a much happier place.

Thirdly I love the work of Atul Gawande, the US surgeon who wrote the books *Checklist Manifesto*, *Complications* and *Better* which are basically a reflective diary of a surgeon's practice. All of these have lots of learnings.

A book I am reading now is about Toyota and the management principles in Toyota. It's called *Toyota Kata* written by Mike Rother and that's all about how Toyota became a successful business based upon their management principles.

The great thing about reading is that you can randomly open a book at one page, read that one page and it will stimulate a whole wave of reflection, new ideas and excitement. When you strip it right back, reading is probably one of the most fundamental and important skills that we will ever learn in life.

Are there any key principles that you try to follow every day? What things do you hold close to you that you think are important?

James: I guess there are a few, James. The first one we all know because we were taught it from when we were kids is to simply "try your best". Steve Peters taught me that a barometer of success is that "you can't do more than your best" but then Dave Brailsford would add an extra line to say, "yes, and you can decide how hard you work to be your best!" I passionately believe you can't do more than your best, though I think Dave is right; the bigger checkpoint is have you actually worked hard enough to be your best. As a result, I'm always trying to be better today than I was yesterday and so on.

As I have mentioned multiple times now, in the last few years, my other principle is to try and strive for balance. I know that I've got the personality that quite often doesn't have balance; I'm "all in" on something and then I'll let everything else drop. Nowadays, I'm trying to have more balance between my personal and professional life. I know that if I spend too much time doing one thing at the expense of the other, eventually I'll come to a standstill, and I won't function well.

Lastly, is how I can help others. If I can get through the day having done my best, tried to have some balance, and finally, helping others, generally it's been a good day. However, this doesn't always happen!

I think the other big principle, which I am a massive believer in, is reflective practice. The times when I've been at my best or learnt the most, have been the times when I was really committed to engaging in reflective practice. Either through writing to myself and/or working with others to work through things together. The times when I have been at my worst, have been times when I haven't thought about things and reflected properly and honestly. So, the principles that I try and follow every day are underpinned by the process of reflection.

In your opinion, what do you think makes a successful performance nutritionist?

James: The answer is in the name. A performance nutritionist is someone who uses nutrition to improve performance. Although this sounds relatively simple and there's a whole host of work and thought that goes into achieving that, the concept is relatively simple. If you can make someone faster, fitter, stronger or fresher, just by changing what they've eaten, then you're doing your job.

MY REFLECTIONS FROM JAMES'S INTERVIEW

It was great to be able to interview James. James is a researcher, practitioner, and friend who I hold so much respect for. James is one of the reasons I studied nutrition and I would not be where I am in my career without him.

What I love about this interview is James's passion and energy for the industry that we work in. It is clear to read how much motivation he has got to move the industry forward and develop individuals around him.

I think it is also important to consider how James also speaks about work ethic, motivation, and resilience within the industry. Ultimately if you are going to achieve then you are going to have to work hard. If you do not want to work hard then do not moan if you are not working where you think you should be, or want to be.

Finally, James talks about how important it is to have world class communication skills but also the ability to coach. I really liked how he simplifies our industry into people who coach. We learn the science and the research and then it is down to us to be able to coach the athlete to the best of our ability to improve their performance.

CONCLUSION:
HOW TO STAND OUT FROM THE CROWD

Before I wrap up this book, I wanted to share with you the Trust Equation, which is used a lot in leadership and management by David Maister, the author of *The Trusted Advisor*. It was taught to me by Professor Graeme Close during my PhD. Graeme explained the Trust Equation as follows:

Credibility + Reliability + Intimacy / Self-interest.

How credible are you, how reliable are you and how intimate are you in your applied practice?

Score yourself out of 10 on each of these and then divide the total score by your self-interest score (also out of 10).

During one of my final PhD meetings before I submitted my thesis, Graeme explained to me how in our careers we should be aiming for a 10 + 10 + 10 for credibility, reliability and intimacy respectively, divided by a "low" self-interest score. You might be thinking why are we not aiming for zero in self-interest instead of low, and this is a valid question. However, in my opinion you will always have a degree of self-interest in the role, otherwise your passion to do the role will not be there. As Eddie Hearn (Matchroom Sport) says, "No Passion, No Point".

To be open and transparent, below are two examples of how I have graded myself against the Trust Equation. When I started my career at Widnes Vikings Rugby League my trust score was: 4 + 4 + 5 / 9 = 1.4.

To be brutally honest, when I worked at Widnes at the start of my career, I loved the role, but I almost loved the role so much that my ego and self-interest got in the way of the delivery of my work. Although I delivered well in this role, I reflect on this 12-month period in my career and wish I had remained humble and concentrated more on reading and becoming more credible, rather than promoting on social media that I was wearing the tracksuit day to day!

The older I have got and the more mature I have become, the more my trust score has improved. My trust score now looks something like this: 7 + 8 + 8 / 4 = 5.7.

What has changed during the last six years of my career? I have focused more on reading the scientific literature, focusing on the task at hand instead of getting distracted, becoming more strategic, improving my communication skills, my awareness, and finally the ability to flex my style in different situations. In turn, this has improved my credibility, reliability and intimacy for the better and allowed my self-interest to gradually decrease. Don't get me wrong, I am still very proud to be working with the organisation and athletes that I do, but the focus is now on development and progression rather than building an ego!

Learning from lessons is very important as nutritionists and I hope you have enjoyed the interviews and the nuggets in this book as much as I've enjoyed recording them. Having personally spoken to each nutritionist for 45–60 minutes, asking them the questions, transcribing their interviews, and then pulling out my key takeaways from each chapter, I can hand on heart say that I have learnt and taken content from all 10 practitioners which I have already started to apply or will apply in my own career and practice.

What I have enjoyed the most through this process is how honest and open each person has been about their journey and path through their unique careers to date. In my opinion, it's something that the nutrition circle does very well. As an industry we are willing to help others out and support each other on our journeys. This is exactly why I wanted to do this book in the first place: to tease out the lessons and advice from others in the industry to see where you and I can learn from them to improve our own practice.

At the start of the book, I said we would deep dive into the lives of successful practitioners currently working in the nutrition space. If like me you have read this book with an open mind and a willingness to learn from others, then I am confident when you reflect on your own path and practice that you will change, tweak and improve things for the better moving forward. For example, you may begin to practice "deep focus" and concentrate a little more on the task at hand instead of getting distracted, or you may make a real effort to be a genuinely nice person as Dr Daniel Martin said in his chapter, or if like me you took a lot from James Morton's interview, you will either continue to work with your mentor or seek a mentor and begin working with them.

What has been humbling about this book is that each one of the interviewees, to some degree, did not actually think they were that successful. However, I would disagree. To work where they work, with professional and elite level athletes, is a success in my opinion. Whether that is the Australian Cycling Team (Jill Leckey), Team Sky cycling team (Professor James Morton), Tottenham Hotspur Football Club (Hannah Sheridan), Professional Jockeys Association (Dr Daniel Martin) or Munster Rugby (Emma Tester), these are all successful careers and careers I know many other practitioners would be extremely proud of.

JAMES'S TOP 15 TIPS

As the author of this book, I wanted to provide my own top tips for anyone wanting to work in the nutrition industry or looking to improve their own practice. This list could go on and on, however I have pulled out 15 of the key areas to start on. This is what I have learnt during my early career to date, from both the academic and practitioner space.

1. BE RESILIENT
You will get something wrong, you will be late, you will forget to do something, and you do not know everything. This is fine. The key thing is how you take the feedback and improve moving forward.

2. ENJOY THE LESSONS
If you get something wrong and learn from it then it is not a mistake. It is a lesson.

3. FACT OR OPINION?
Always find out the facts first and bin the opinions. I have been involved in too many conversations where people say, "I think the food is poor, I don't think the team like this, blah blah blah". Ask the person, is what you're about to tell me fact or is it your opinion?

4. THE WHOLE WORLD EATS FOOD!
Everyone in the world eats food and therefore everyone in the world will have an opinion on it. Face it with a smile, embrace it and use it to have a richer conversation with that person.

5. EXPECTATION OF ATHLETE KNOWLEDGE
Do not expect athletes to know as much as you do about nutrition. They have not studied a degree, master's or PhD in it and therefore may not understand some of the basic principles of our industry. It is down to you to coach them to understand it and understand it properly.

Likewise, some athletes do know a lot about nutrition, and these can be wonderful conversations. Enjoy them but also do not try to bluff your way through them. If they ask you a question and you are not confident with the answer, then say so. You will get more respect by saying, "I'm sorry, I have not read enough in this area yet, let me go and read the literature and come back to you tomorrow".

6. QUICKLY BECOME SOMEONE WHO LOVES TO READ
As Professors James Morton and Graeme Close used to always say to me, "Read the literature, read it again and then read some more of it. Remember we are researchers first, practitioners second".

7. LEARN HOW TO BE A GREAT COACH

Become a better coach. We are in the coaching industry, and it is down to us to coach the athletes to be better informed about how nutrition can improve performance. This will include being a brilliant communicator both in person and remotely. Think about how you currently deliver your education and check and challenge yourself to be able to do it better. I went on a brilliant course called "High Performance Presentations" by Dale Carnegie. It taught me all about how to better communicate and especially how to use hand gestures to embed your point.

8. AS THE NEW ZEALAND ALL BLACKS (RUGBY TEAM) SAY... DON'T BE A D**K HEAD.

Being a good person will really go a long way in our industry. Be polite, smile and respect all of those around you.

9. BE COMFORTABLE IN ASKING

Do not be afraid to reach out and ask for advice, help or support.

10. VOLUNTEER

Volunteer and embrace it. We have all been there and you are no different. Take any opportunities you can to get hands-on experience with athletes. This includes if you are at university; take part in research studies and assist PhD students. You will learn so much from this.

11. BECOME A DEAL MASTER

Learn how to secure partnerships and deals with external providers. This will be key to allowing you to have a big impact and quickly.

12. PICK THE LOW HANGING FRUIT FIRST

What areas of delivery will have the biggest impact for you, but more importantly quickly? Forget trying to implement a creatine intake strategy if your players don't understand how to fuel correctly for training!

13. WHAT IS YOUR USP (UNIQUE SELLING POINT)?

Think about what makes you different to everyone else. If there is nothing, then you need to work on this now and start to stand out from the crowd. Maybe you need a mentor to help you with this?

14. LEARN THE DUNNING KRUGER MODEL

Learn the Dunning Kruger model and always check in with yourself to see where you are on the curve! Where possible you are trying to remain as far away as possible from the Peak of "Mount Stupid" phase!!

15. ENJOY BEING PART OF A MULTIDISCIPLINARY TEAM

Enjoy working as part of a multidisciplinary team. You will have fantastic conversations with practitioners from other disciplines and quite often they will see things through a different lens to you which will improve your practice.

FIND OUT MORE ABOUT MOREHEN PERFORMANCE MENTORSHIP

"Helping practitioners and researchers to develop individually, increasing their value, growth and worth through experiences, exposures, knowledge, networks and applied skills"

I hope you have benefited from my tips and the tips of those whom I have interviewed for this book. What I also want to ensure is that you have the right support and advice going forward in your career. That's where I can help you further.

WHAT DOES THE MENTORSHIP INVOLVE?
This programme will support and guide you to identify what success looks like for you, what barriers are in your way currently and how to overcome them and work through a framework and programme together to create impact for your work and success in your career.

As it is individualised, this is a dynamic process that will adapt and develop as you grow and develop yourself. The whole process is defined by you, and delivered by you with my support, to ensure you hit the targets and goals you have along what will be a great journey.

HOW WILL THE PROGRAMME WORK?

Regular coaching calls will allow us to further develop your skills and knowledge, be creative in how we solve issues, and allow you to hit your goals and targets set out at the start of the programme.

Each month will include:

- A 45–60 min coaching call
- Feedback notes supported with actions for both you and me
- Provision of key materials, documents and research related to and aligned to your needs
- Access to my experience and knowledge over the last eight years of working in high-performance sport
- Access to my key contacts at many sport supplement and sports food companies

There will also be:

- A quarterly review for us both to reflect on your progress and to refine your objectives and plans moving forward
- The option to become part of a private WhatsApp group to network, share and discuss with other like-minded individuals

PRAISE FOR MOREHEN PERFORMANCE MENTORSHIP

Here are some words from a few of my mentees about what it's like working with me:

Mentee 1 – Second year sport and exercise nutrition undergraduate student transitioning into third year of their course

> "I feel like I've achieved so much already! Within days of my mentorship starting, he approached me with a paid opportunity to work with Olympic athletes.

> "I've had professional meetings with reputable figures in the industry and with James's guidance I've been able to present my thoughts and ideas on possible nutritional strategies to consider. A mentorship like this does not come without its obstacles. What's great about James is, he asks me questions that allow me to really dissect and critically evaluate for myself.

> "James helps me develop my skills to become a better practitioner. He sets me tasks to complete that will help with my development, whether that be reading up on specific sports nutrition for my work experience

or contacting people in my network to gain potential clients. During the calls, I feel like I'm speaking to a long-term friend and always feel comfortable saying anything to him.

"Starting my mentorship with James has truly been the best decision I've made! So much has happened in so little time and I'm excited to see what's to come. Thanks James!"

Mentee 2 – Applied placement student in a football club

"In terms of mentorship and guidance I couldn't recommend James any higher, he's been a constant source of knowledge and experience, with a firm grasp of the many practical applications that surround it. Allowing me to see the nutrition world from his perspective has been nothing short of revolutionary in terms of the way I approach my work and the challenges this work entails. He consistently challenges your ideas and perspective in a manner underpinned by a polite and upbeat approach that only serves to encourage you to improve. I have no doubt that the ideas he's encouraged me to make and the concepts he's challenged me to understand have helped build the foundations of a successful career in the evolving world of nutrition."

Mentee 3 – Currently working in Ireland with professional Gaelic football players

"It has been a great experience to link in with James while progressing my career as a performance nutritionist. James's experience of working in elite level sport has been invaluable to me. Would definitely recommend James to anyone looking to gain practical and innovative nutritional strategies for team success."

Mentee 4 – Graduate from sport nutrition master's course

"Being mentored by James has been a great step in the right direction for me. He has helped me to develop as a person as well as in my nutrition practice. He has put me in touch with contacts and helped me to start taking on independent clients, such as a professional footballer. I am looking forward to continuing to work with him, and what the future will hold."

Mentee 5 – Sports nutritionist in France

"About a year ago, I started working with elite athletes preparing for the Winter Olympics. I decided to join James's programme and I'm so glad I did.

"James's expertise at an elite level, across many different sports, has been absolutely invaluable. As well as helping with the nutrition strategy itself, every idea and suggestion is underpinned by his understanding of how that can realistically be applied in the field and on competition days, as well as the mentality of the coaches and athletes. It is that ability to not just translate the latest research into applied practice, but fully integrate the two, that makes his advice so valuable.

"Since working with James, I have much more confidence in my own ability. I also have the reassurance that if I don't know something or am struggling to find an answer to a problem, James is only a phone call away. Having that support has demonstrably increased my confidence when talking to athletes, coaches and other stakeholders at all levels, which has undoubtedly made me a more effective practitioner.

"In the few months that I have been working with James, I (we) have achieved amazing results with athletes that I previously would not have had the confidence to work with, and as a direct result of James's input, I gained an offer to work even more closely with national level teams on an ongoing basis. We have also set long-term goals and having those to work towards, as well as knowing that we always have another call scheduled, has really helped me maintain focus, motivation and productivity – no mean feat when self-employed and working from home in the middle of a pandemic!

"To put it simply, joining James's mentorship programme is the best business investment I have made since graduating as a nutritionist."

KEEP IN TOUCH

To get involved with the mentorship programme, please reach out to me at:

Website: morehenperformance.com
Email: morehenperformanceltd@gmail.com

To follow me and see more of what I do in the research, academic and applied world, please follow me at:

Twitter: @James_Morehen
Instagram: MorehenPerformance

Finally, thank you so much for your support with this project. I have already started my research for my second book, so make sure you sign up to get the details.

https://morehenperformance.com/pages/the-performance-nutritionist

REFERENCES

Daring Greatly: How the Courage to Be Vulnerable Transforms the Way We Live, Love, Parent, and Lead, Brené Brown

Case Study: Resumption of Eumenorrhea in Parallel With High Training Load After 4 Years of Menstrual Dysfunction: A 5-year Follow-Up of an Elite Female Cyclist, Jose L. Areta, International Journal of Sport Nutrition and Exercise Metabolism, Feb 27 2020;1–6

Navy Seal Admiral William H. McRaven https://www.youtube.com/watch?v=mMEqor97T_k

The Chimp Paradox: The Mind Management Programme for Confidence, Success and Happiness, Professor Steve Peters

Dare to Lead: Brave Work. Tough Conversations. Whole Hearts, Brené Brown

The Culture Code: The Secrets of Highly Successful Groups, Daniel Coyle

Deep Work: Rules for Focused Success in a Distracted World, Cal Newport

BOSH! Simple Recipes, Amazing Food, All Plants, Henry Firth and Ian Theasby

A Promised Land, Barack Obama

Atomic Habits: An Easy and Proven Way to Build Good Habits and Break Bad Ones, James Clear

Eddie Hearn, Matchroom Sport, podcast "No Passion, No Point" https://podcasts.apple.com/gb/podcast/eddie-hearn-no-passion-no-point/id1465770394

The Complete Guide to Sports Nutrition, Anita Bean

Can't Hurt Me: Master Your Mind and Defy the Odds, David Goggins

Hostage at the Table: How Leaders Can Overcome Conflict, Influence Others, and Raise Performance, George Kohlrieser

The Body Keeps the Score: Mind, Brain and Body in the Transformation of Trauma, Bessel van der Kolk

The Power of Habit: Why We Do What We Do, and How to Change, Charles Duhigg

A brief introduction to the COM-B Model of behaviour and the PRIME Theory of motivation, Robert West and Susan Michie, available at https://discovery.ucl.ac.uk/id/eprint/10095639/1/WW04E6.2.pdf

The Infinite Game: How Great Businesses Achieve Long-lasting Success, Simon Sinek

Score Takes Care of Itself: My Philosophy of Leadership, Bill Walsh

How to Win Friends and Influence People, Dale Carnegie

Checklist Manifesto: How to Get Things Right, Atul Gawande

Toyota Kata: Managing People for Improvement, Adaptiveness and Superior Results, Mike Rother

The Trusted Advisor: 20th Anniversary Edition, David H. Maister, Charles H. Green & Robert M. Galford

Unskilled and Unaware of It: How Difficulties in Recognizing One's Own Incompetence Lead to Inflated Self-Assessments, Justin Kruger and David Dunning, Journal of Personality and Social Psychology, Dec 1999;77(6):1121–34

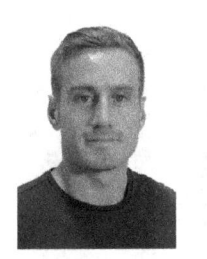

ABOUT THE AUTHOR

Prior to university James spent three years travelling across Southeast Asia and teaching snowboarding in Canada. At the age of 21 he decided to stop travelling and embarked on a nine-year academic career at Liverpool John Moores University within the Research Institute for Sport and Exercise Sciences. Here he completed his undergraduate degree in Sport and Exercise Science and his Master's in Sports Physiology. James then completed his PhD titled: Growing, building and repairing elite rugby players: nutritional and energetic considerations.

Throughout his studies, his applied work with elite sport included professional athletes from football, rugby, boxing, motorsport, combat sports, golf as well as global companies such as IKEA, Credit Suisse and HSBC Global.

James is proudly registered with the Sport and Exercise Nutrition Register as a high-performance practitioner and, outside of working with elite athletes, enjoys reviewing the current literature, presenting at universities, mentoring others in the industry and running his own business, Morehen Performance Ltd.

In his spare time James enjoys relaxing with his partner Nura, his dog Sunny and his family.

CPSIA information can be obtained
at www.ICGtesting.com
Printed in the USA
BVHW040847081221
623507BV00010B/230